Dreams,
Images, and
Fantasy

UNIVERSITY OF ILLINOIS PRESS Urbana Chicago London

Dreams,
Images, and
Fantasy:
A Semantic
Differential
Casebook

C. SCOTT MOSS

To Joel, Julie, and Kevin — my "dreams" of the future.

CONTENTS

FOREWORD

Charles E. Osgood

In the decade or so since publication of *The Measurement of Meaning* there has been a rash of literature involving the semantic differential technique in one way or another. A fairly up-to-date bibliography (see Snider and Osgood, 1969) lists some 1,500 titles, but this is by no means exhaustive. A rather sizable portion of this literature comes from the general area of personality, clinical psychology, and psychotherapy. In scanning a sample of this material in preparation of the source book referred to above, it became painfully obvious that much of it was either shoddily done or consisted of one-shot affairs by the authors concerned — or both. Those who have combined methodological sophistication about the technique with persistence in the pursuit of a significant problem can be counted on the fingers of one hand, or at most both. One of these is the author of this book.

C. Scott Moss encountered the semantic differential technique early in his — and its — career. He was, I am proud to say, one of my first Ph.D. advisees, soon after I came to the University of Illinois in 1949. While George Suci, Percy Tannenbaum, and I were struggling with the methodology itself as a way of measuring at least some aspects of meaning (the affective components, it now appears), Scott was busily applying an early form to the study of dream symbolism in several of his patients — and in the process providing one of the first tests of the validity of the technique. His doctoral thesis was not the end, but rather the beginning of an exploration into the nature of dreams, armed with hypnosis as a clinical tool and the semantic differential as a method of measurement.

Not being a clinician myself — my only excursion into this important but obscure domain being a blind analysis of a case of multiple personality ("The Three Faces of Eve") with Zella Luria — I cannot speak to the clinical sophistication of the author of this book or to its potential contribution in this field. Nevertheless, even as a rank outsider I am impressed by the way clinical sensitivities and insights are combined with quantitative measurements of meanings in the several case studies reported here. I have the opinion (based primarily on being a member of many thesis committees for clinical students!) that the one is often sacrificed for the other. Nor can I comment with any authority on the prospects for intensive, time-limited hypnotherapy, although the social need for such therapy, extending both the numbers and kinds of patients who can be effectively treated, is obvious. Should the semantic differential technique prove to be a sufficiently valid and sensitive reflector of what is going on in patients' minds, one can imagine a coupling of it to modern computer technology which might vastly extend the efficiency of clinical practice. But this is merely a little dream of my own.

Although in this book, as in most applications of the semantic differential technique in psychotherapy, the semantic data are used primarily as a *test* or validation of clinical intuitions, one wonders to what extent such data could serve as a *source* of clinical hypotheses. To what extent could the therapist use the meanings of critical concepts, their distances and clusterings, their polarizations, and the changes in these measures as the source of insights into the nature of the patient's disorder? Into the effects of therapy? Into prognosis as well as diagnosis? In a sense, this is exactly what Zella Luria and I were trying to do — of necessity — in our blind analysis of "The Three Faces of Eve." As a matter of fact, we suggested that the third personality which evolved in therapy ("Jane") was probably a role being played and was not a successful resolution of the case — which happened to prove true in this instance.

But what happens when semantic differential data conflict with clinical judgment? I am sure that today therapists would place much more confidence in their clinical intuitions — which, after all, are nested (however vaguely) in the intimate matrix of close personal interactions and observations — than in the posturings of what, after all, are merely arrays of checkmarks on scales. Yet there is a sense in which these little checkmarks are closer to the patient's mind than a therapist can ever be. So the basis for trust may change in time, if this technique's validity can be clearly demonstrated.

The high point of this book for me, at least, is the very fine chapter on the theory of symbolism in dreams. Here, with the reader's mind already bubbling with case studies and experiments on dream symbolism, Moss draws — out of the classic observations on dreams, out of mediation learning theory, and out of his own fertile intuitions — an integrative theoretical framework within which existing evidence, including his own, on the nature of dream-work seems to fit like a hand in a tailor-made glove. The dynamics of motivational conflict between the need to express (the latent content) and the need to repress (the disguising manifest content) and the dynamics of cognitive interaction, among the affective and denotative features of the symbol and what is symbolized, are worked into a very convincing theoretical framework. It is more than a theory of dream symbolism, however, carrying as it does implications for waking symbolism, the process of metaphor-making, and the nature of aesthetics generally.

C. Scott Moss is to be congratulated for giving us a book that contributes significantly to the theory of meaning as well as to the practice of psychotherapy.

PREFACE

At this juncture, I am not the advocate of any particular "school" in psychotherapy. I am an eclectic. I was brought up in a quasi-psychoanalytic orientation, and I basically owe my allegiance to learning theory, but I was also tainted and enthralled by several early clinical supervisors, specifically L. A. Pennington and Jack Watkins, who favored hypnotherapy. In this book I take the occasion to indulge myself in whatever clinical insights may have derived from my 20 years of dealing with patients in hypnosis, using the semantic differential as the basic objective measuring tool in my clinical bag.

I would be remiss not to mention the influence which Charles Osgood had on my professional development. I went into clinical psychology because I had a strong motivation to help others, and by the third graduate year, I still had little interest in academic psychology and research. I ended up doing my dissertation with "Charlie" and I never worked so hard for a year and a half as I did for him; but out of this came a new-won respect for research which changed the future course of my professional life. He personified perfection and he demanded this quality from his subordinates. From that time on, I was a clinical (and later a community) psychologist with a strong personal interest in applied research. I had learned that good research is definitely a service to the practicing psychologist.

There are a number of other people who deserve mention, such as my colleague, Julian Rappaport, who made several valuable comments about the manuscript. Let me also single out my wife, Bette, who more than anyone else has promoted my time for writing, performed a host of secretarial functions, and occasionally protected me from the many demands of my three charming children and our affectionate white Boxer dog.

C. Scott Moss
Urbana, Illinois
1970

Dreams,
Images, and
Fantasy

ONE   Introduction

The mental health program of the United States is confronted by
a rapidly developing crisis. The public's demand for services already exceeds the availability of professional manpower to de-
liver them. The advent of Medicare and Medicaid — with the
sudden eligibility of 35,000,000 aged and indigent Americans —
can only exacerbate an already serious problem. One obvious
remedy would be to greatly accelerate the training of traditional
mental health professional disciplines, but this provides no immediate solution and present plans in this regard are quite inadequate. A second possible solution is the increased utilization of
nonprofessional, subprofessional, and allied professional sources
of manpower; however, while some imaginative exploratory projects are underway in this area, the established professional orga-
nizations have not enthusiastically endorsed this alternative. A
third approach is to maximize employment of available mental
health professional resources through more efficient and effective
practices. There is little scientifically established evidence to support the present definition of roles, functions, and services.

This book will address itself to a relatively restricted aspect of
one part of the problem of reformulating the professional treatment role, namely, stressing an intensive, time-limited, crisis-oriented psychotherapy and, most specifically, the uses of hypnosis
as a facilitant to brief psychotherapy. With few exceptions, psy-

chiatrists and psychologists engaged in outpatient treatment provide long-term psychotherapy (an average well in excess of 200 hours per patient over an 18-month to three-year period). This approach has two major limitations: (1) the inordinate duration and (2) the exclusion of "unsophisticated people," particularly the culturally and economically deprived. Most experienced therapists are, therefore, available only to a small economically privileged segment of society, at an exorbitant cost in time and money, and with the added stipulation that patients be verbally facile, possessed of an unusual introspective capacity, and skilled in the manipulation of abstract concepts. It is estimated that three-quarters of the applicants for treatment of emotional disorders come from lower- or lower-middle-class socio-economic backgrounds even at the present time. This proportion will certainly increase with Medicare and Medicaid resulting in a continuing and increasing referral to state mental hospitals and other public facilities of a highly disproportionate number of the economically and culturally deprived.

Two other factors are acting to radically alter the pattern of mental health services in the United States in the immediate future: (1) the widespread increase of group health insurance, including coverage for the treatment of psychiatric disorders, particularly among union members who are not economically deprived but who do generally lack the capacity for trained introspection, and (2) commitment of the national mental health program to a shift in the locus of treatment from isolated state mental hospitals to community-based programs through the construction during the next two decades of several thousand comprehensive community mental health centers (this is number-one priority of the National Institute of Mental Health, USPHS). It is hoped that this program will result in much more than a change in locus, viz., the stimulation of creative innovations in the character of community mental health services.

Time-limited psychotherapy is known by various terms, including confrontation technique, brief psychotherapy, short-term dynamic psychotherapy, short-term therapy, behavioral therapy, recompensation therapy, crisis resolution, precipitating stress as a focus in psychotherapy, and supportive care program. It is currently beginning to be applied to numerous psychiatric and psychologic problems. There is a rapidly growing literature offering conceptual formulations of stress, crisis intervention, the use of time-limited services, and their relevance for community mental health policy and preventive services (Bellak and Small, 1965; Caplan, 1964; Parad, 1965; Phillips and Wiener, 1966; Wolberg, 1965). Emergency or crisis-oriented treatments are geared to a focused and prompt response to requests for service. Professional skills are immediately made available in periods of crisis when the vulnerability of patients and the condition of problems render them most amenable to change. A major attraction of hypnosis to professional personnel has always been the promise of appreciably reducing the extended duration of psychotherapy, and it would appear to offer attractive advantages as a relatively brief form of psychotherapy; however, this is a promise that in the past has often been made but seldom met.

Through the centuries the troubled person has always sought refuge from the threatening environment with some individual whom he believed to possess special and often supernatural powers. In this protective environment, he was trained and encouraged to take his place back in the world. In ancient Greece, a troubled person was treated with rest, suggestion, diet, baths, massage, exercise, and discussed his problems with a friendly philosopher or was instructed to act out his problem in dramatics. In severe cases, it is reputed that an electric eel might even be applied to his forehead. Such humane and understanding treatment was a singular exception. Historically, man has always shared his world with a variety of demons, ghosts, goblins, devils, and spirits to whom he assigned responsibility for his behavior and destiny. The natural treatment regimen under the circumstances was some form of exorcism of evil involving the practice of magic. Strangely enough, we find the origin of the psychological point of view in a rather unexpected place — in the study of hypnosis. Anton Mesmer (1734–1815) is often characterized as the first of the modern-day psychotherapists. Through use of magnetic fluids, Mesmer was able to induce bizarre behavior (convulsions or crises) and to actually effect cures. Suggestion has really been a basic therapeutic technique for thousands of years. For what a person believes in quite literally determines reality for him. Change a person's attitudes and you alter his perception of the world about him. This is the essence of most therapies.

Hypnotherapy need not be simply an abbreviated version of traditional long-term psychotherapy (e.g., an adjunctive technique), nor need be limited to persons who are temperamentally introspective, verbally fluent, and can think conceptually. Hypnotherapy as practiced here is an emotionally corrective therapeutic experience. It frees fantasy and imagination, allowing access to preconscious and unconscious content, and it encourages memorial reversion, so that patients can move flexibly along the time continuum, living and re-experiencing the past and comparing and contrasting past with present perceptions, emotions, and experiences. The intensity of mental imagery solicited through hypnosis encourages a direct reconditioning process. It is also a procedure that largely relieves the therapist of the need for involved interpretations, since hypnotically induced experiences are both revelationary and convincing. Contrary to popular opinion, effective hypnotherapy does not require a high level of susceptibility, so that benefit can be derived by patients possessed of even modest suggestibility (75 percent of the population). Similarly, effective hypnotherapy should be essentially problem- and not symptom-oriented, even though the danger of symptom removal is a tenet of psychoanalytic faith and not a proven fact. As a form of brief psychotherapy it will be concerned much more with precipitating (recent) than predisposing (historical or childhood psychogenic) factors, and treatment objectives will necessarily be circumscribed. The basic premise underlying the crisis intervention approach is that the successful resolution of even one major, immediate problem can lead to the re-establishment of a patient's psychological equilibrium.

The book includes a well-considered concern with methods of objective assessment and evaluation of this mode of treatment. Since treatment is time-limited and goals are quite specific, usually involving an alteration in presenting complaints combined with a long-term followup (to see if changes are sustained), brief psychotherapy lends itself to an easier assessment than more extended forms of psychotherapy. Especial emphasis will be placed on clinical research trends involving the semantic differential (Osgood et al., 1957), not only in the evaluation of brief crisis-oriented psychotherapy but in a variety of other contexts as well.

The semantic differential is not a particular test but rather a highly generalizable operation of measurement which can be adapted to specific research problems. Its originator, Charles Osgood, postulates a geometrical model in the form of a semantic space defined by logical opposites. Factor analysis was used to identify the independent dimensions of this space, representing the ways human beings make affective meaning judgments. Three factors, evaluation, potency, and activity, account for 50 percent of the total variance in how people make meaningful judgments, of which the evaluation dimension accounts for two-thirds. The generality of this factor structure was further tested by varying subject populations, concepts judged, type of judgmental situation, and the factoring method used in analyzing data.

The measuring operation or semantic differential can be described as follows. Adjectives are identified as representative of these three major dimensions along which affective meaningful processes vary; these have a high coverage of meaning on one factor and negligible amount on the others. These opposites are used to define the ends of seven-point scales. In practice, an individual judges a particular concept against a set of these scales.

Judgments result in the successive allocation of a concept to a point in multidimensional space. In this manner, change in the meaning of a concept over time, the subtle differences between two or more concepts, and individual differences in the meaning of a single concept may be quantitatively represented.

Osgood and other investigators have, of course, had a continuing interest in the attempt to identify what they have referred to as the basic dimensions of meaning in language behavior. In the attempt to purify the factor structure and to isolate more sensitive scales to represent each factor, investigations have continued in which adjectives, concepts, subject populations, and methods of factor analysis have been varied. People working with the semantic differential have been increasingly interested in the personality and psychotherapy area. Although there are hundreds of "personality tests" available, there does not seem to be any standardized way of simply describing (and hence accurately communicating) the individual personality. "Personality" can be regarded as essentially a meaningful construct developed out of interpersonal interactions, and therefore the general techniques of semantic measurement should be applicable. And it is usually the connotative meaning ("feeling tone") rather than the denotative meaning (name, physical characteristics, etc.) of the person in which there is interest.

The earliest study of changes in meaning experienced by patients in psychotherapy using the semantic differential technique was performed by O. H. Mowrer (1953). He had two patients, suffering from agoraphobia, judge eight concepts (ME, MOTHER, FATHER, BABY, LADY, GOD, SIN, and FRAUD) at the beginning, middle, and termination of psychotherapy. He interpreted the results as substantiating his theoretical position that the neurotic is typically a person who represses his own self-critical faculty (conscience). A second early application of the differential to investigate semantic changes in psychotherapy was done by Moss (1953). He obtained ratings of concepts from two patients at several points during the course of therapy. An innovation which Moss introduced was to obtain differential ratings under the hypnotic state which, as a presumed index of "unconscious" meanings, could be compared with ratings made in the waking state, as an index of "conscious" meanings. Obtained data indicated a wide discrepancy between waking and hypnotic ratings at the beginning of therapy and a significant reduction as treatment progressed. Briefly, these results were interpreted to mean that areas of neurotic conflict within the personality are characterized by dissociation such that different levels of meaning, conscious and unconscious, coexist, and that as conflict is resolved, there is integration of these originally discrepant levels.

An approach to the problem of an accurate characterization of patient personality was next undertaken by the semantic analysis of "The Three Faces of Eve." On the basis of the differentials given to the three aspects of this personality, Osgood and Luria (1954) questioned whether the emergent personality, Jane, was a successful resolution of therapy. This doubt was later verified when it was found that Jane was simply Eve Black playing the role of a person acceptable to the therapist. The original clue was that the semantic structure derived from Jane's ratings was collapsed or oversimplified; that is, there was a reduction in discrimination so that it became almost entirely evaluative in nature. Evidence indicates that when people role-play, there is a detectable simplification of the semantic structure.

Z. Luria (1959) checked a number of hypotheses concerning the nature of meaning changes of patients in psychotherapy. She found, for example, that prospective therapy subjects can be discriminated from normals on the basis of their relative devaluation of SELF and PARENT concepts. Somewhat surprisingly, therapy resulted in an increase in positive attitude toward SELF but not toward the parents. Her study highlights the basic question of the intelligent selection of concepts more relevant or sensitive to changes expected with psychotherapy. There have been, of course, many studies on psychotherapy and the semantic differential since these early ones.

This book features a special variant of psychotherapy that might be called "hypnosymbolic treatment," which is a natural extension and clinical application of techniques described in the book, *The Hypnotic Investigation of Dreams* (Moss, 1967b). Specifically, the present book begins with a reprint of a paper on the experimental paradigms for the investigation of hypnotic dreaming, which sets the tone and gives the reader insight into the methodology of semantic differential measurement. Next is an intensive case study involving the hypnotic interpretation of nocturnal dreams, with a special emphasis on the mode of symbolic representations and also an attempt to objectively assess the changes in the subject throughout therapy. The chapter which follows involves a two-fold effort to test the capacity of hypnotic subjects to interpret the symbols generated by others; and the fifth chapter involves the alteration of social attitudes toward the Negro and is a test of Osgood's "congruity hypothesis" using hypnosis. The last investigation has to do with a test of the reliability of the Szondi categories. This is the only study that does not deal with hypnosis, but was included on the basis that it does deal with projection which is the essense of dreaming.

The final chapter in Part I (Experimental Results) follows a redefining of terms and hypotheses in testable form, showing how the phenomena of symbolism can be incorporated into Osgood's (1953) mediation theory of behavior, which was formulated to provide a theoretical framework for research into the complex intervening process of *meaning* in the human organism.

The second part of the book (Clinical Studies) contains a trilogy of representative case studies. The first report is of symptomatic relief of a case of wartime neurosis; the second study is a detailed account of the psychotherapy of one female patient — a treatment failure — but it is the stimulus for discussion of the genetics and dynamics of hysteria; the third report is a study of a woman suffering from confused sexual identity. Chapter Nine includes a verbatim account of the hypnotherapy of a patient suffering an acute phobic reaction; the results are again substantiated by the patient's semantic differential ratings.

The last chapter provides a review of the fundamental factors which go into a hypnosymbolic technique of dealing therapeutically with a person's dreams, and it attempts to summarize the basic principles derived from many years of experience with the method.

PART I   EXPERIMENTAL RESULTS

TWO

Experimental Paradigms for the Hypnotic Investigation of Dream Symbolism[1]

The process of symbolization has been both the most intriguing and controversial aspect of the rich fabric of theory advanced by psychoanalysis and, unfortunately, the most resistant to scientific exploration. This paper will outline a variety of experimental approaches to the investigation of dream symbolism through innovations in hypnotic technique. The value of hypnosis in dream research is that it seemingly provides access to the symbol-translating mechanism. For instance, recall of forgotten dream elements can be facilitated, some subjects are able to "dream" upon command, and others demonstrate an increased capacity to interpret symbolic materials (Erickson and Kubie, 1938, 1940; Farber and Fisher, 1943; Rapaport, 1951). The principal measuring instrument employed throughout these studies was the semantic differential, a method specifically designed to provide an objective measurement of the connotative (feeling) aspect of meaning.

In an early experiment (Moss, 1957a), an attempt was made to test the psychoanalytic idea of dream symbol disguise by translating it into the operationally defined concept of *semantic distance*. Ordinarily choice of a symbol should be determined by the similarity of mediational processes between a potential symbol and the latent content to be represented. However, according

[1] Reprinted by permission from *International Journal of Clinical and Experimental Hypnosis*, 9, no. 3 (July, 1961): 105–117.

to Freud, anxiety-stimulating latent content results in the choice of symbols that are semantically distant; a symbol that is semantically distant from the latent content becomes unintelligible and may be said to be disguised.

Seventy-six dreams of a single patient in psychotherapy over a year were intensively studied. A form of the semantic differential was used to measure the distance between symbol and latent content when the covert content was anxiety-arousing and when it was not. In operational terms, disguise would be indicated by a relative increase in semantic distance coincident with anxiety.

Identification of the meaning of dream symbols used by the patient-subject was a primary problem, and reliance upon conventional methods of interpretation was supplemented by training the patient to interpret his own dreams under hypnosis. The patient free-associated to the dream elements, first in the waking and then in the hypnotic state, in order to identify the latent content. Associative material obtained in hypnosis was invariably centrally related to the meaning of the dream.

The following dream demonstrates the highly meaningful nature of the patient's dreams and his facility in dream interpretation.

The patient and his wife were going on an ocean voyage. They found the gangplank steep and lined with girls. On deck the captain inquired whether the patient had a newspaper. When the patient replied that he did not, the captain assured him that he'd find one in his cabin. The patient next traveled slowly down a spiral slide and found himself seated in the dining room. There he refused an offer of hamburgers. He was suddenly ashore again, standing beside a convertible. A voice said, "Tell your uncle he is holding up the works."

Waking associations. The dream was essentially without meaning to the patient. The predominant emotion was apprehension. The significant associations were as follows. *Water*: the patient had long suffered a mild aquaphobia. *Voyage*: his only sea voyage was in military service. *Hamburgers*: the patient was surprised at his refusal since he liked hamburgers. *Uncle*: a favorite with the patient.

Hypnotic reconstruction. The patient's first association was to *ocean voyage.* "The phrase 'going from the old to the new' enters my mind." He then drew the analogy that therapy is a means of exchanging an old, unsatisfactory adjustment for a new mode and in this sense is like a journey. "I also find myself thinking of the voyage I took in service and how frightened I was." Therapy is therefore initially perceived as "a voyage on dangerous waters." (Later it became apparent that the patient unconsciously associated the awesome, cruel, overpowering quality of water with intense hostile impulses threatening his control and self-esteem.) The next association was to *gangplank*: "I remember how very steep it seemed — it was hard getting aboard. My *wife* being with me meant that this is *our* problem — she's the main reason I'm here." The *line of girls* momentarily thwarted recognition, but the patient then stated quite positively they represented different aspects of the relationship with his wife. To *ship captain* he associated, "Men who are strong and strict, but just — it makes me think of in here, of you, that you will help channel my thoughts into the right direction, also that it will not be an easy job, either." The *newspaper* was explained as a reference to the dreams he had been told to report, i.e., "both are a chronicle of events." "I remember telling you I didn't dream very often and you said 'don't worry about it.' 'Below decks' makes me think of 'below the surface' — dreams come from below the surface when one sleeps, in the cabin or bedroom." The patient interpreted the *slide* as "a roundabout way of reaching a goal," meaning his old inadequate mode of adjustment. "I'm afraid that when the going gets tough, I'll slide back into the old way of thinking." "*Hamburgers* make me think of 'food for thought' — they represent the things we're talking about here, things that are distasteful and I don't want to face or swallow." The *return to shore* was interpreted by the patient as another expression of ambivalence toward therapy, that is, his fear that the content discussed would be unpleasant and he would want to escape. The *convertible*, like the slide, was translated as an old and established but "unsafe" (neurotic) mode of goal attainment. The verbal reference to the *uncle* stimulated recall of a recent statement by the uncle to the effect that the primary defect of the patient was a lack of self-confidence. This remark sensitized the patient to his tendency to be withdrawn from problem situations and made it difficult for him to retreat from therapy, i.e., "This remark keeps me from using the convertible." The three component parts of the dream are thus ambivalence toward therapy, rejection of the situation, but inability to return to the old adjustment.

When the patient presented such a dream, one or more symbols were selected, and he was asked to rate these in the dream context on the differential. The patient would associate to the dream, first in the waking and then in the hypnotic state, in order to establish the latent meaning. Subsequently, in the waking state with complete recall for his dream analysis, the patient rated the identified latent content.

No adequate measure of the anxiety associated with a specific dream symbol was available; however, independent measures (psychological tests and staff ratings) indicated progressive patient improvement over a year's time. In addition, five clinicians agreed in classifying 13 of the patient's dreams as highly anxious ("nightmares"), 11 of which occurred in the first half of therapy. Contrary to psychoanalytic theory, the semantic distances between the mediational processes of dream symbols and things symbolized, as reflected on the differential, were not significantly greater for the first half as compared with the second half of therapy. Thus the hypothesis that dream symbols acquire a disguise function under the impetus of anxiety was not substantiated.

Mature consideration, however, led to the recognition that the semantic differential had definite limitations in detecting the effect of a dream censorship process. While many competent therapists seem agreed that the affective qualities of the dream are usually not subject to distortion, this is the aspect of meaning primarily measured by the differential. Needed was the development of a denotative differential. Since the relationship between symbol and latent content is typically quite tenuous, such a measuring instrument would also have to be extremely sensitive to relatively minute and highly individual aspects of meaning, rather than measuring the common variance among groups of subjects.

A second study used a form of the differential composed of scales designed to measure physical qualities (e.g., large-small, wet-dry, long-short, angular-rounded, etc.); subjects were also instructed to respond to the "physical" rather than the "feeling" characteristics of symbols and things symbolized. Instead of spontaneous night dreams, data this time consisted of hypnotically induced "dreams."

Three normal, psychologically naive subjects were first intensively studied through interview and projective techniques in order to identify areas of personal conflict. They were then induced to "dream" under hypnosis about both pleasant and unpleasant, or anxiety-arousing, personal content. The hypnotic products were typically similar to the autosymbolic phenomena experienced in the transitional hypnagogic state between waking and sleep; while symbols were employed, they appeared relatively poor in multiple meaning.

A female subject's concern regarding a dependency conflict is depicted in this brief, representative "dream."

I was hit by a big truck which came to rest on me. It was very heavy. I appealed to my parents to remove it but they ignored me. I struggled very hard and finally succeeded in pushing it off.

In every instance the subject was instructed to be amnesic for the dream suggestion. At the conclusion of a dream the subject rated selected dream symbols on the differential (e.g., TRUCK). She was next asked to associate to the dream in the waking and hypnotic states in order to clarify and confirm the meaning of the latent content, and to rate this content on the differential (e.g., GUILT RELATED TO MY STRUGGLE FOR INDEPENDENCE).

Ratings of 42 symbols and the corresponding latent content were obtained from 31 anxiety-provoking dreams, while 34 such measurements were obtained from 22 dreams with pleasant content. The average semantic distance under the two conditions for each of the three subjects did not differ significantly. These investigations again failed to support the hypothesized effect of a censorship mechanism; the results of both studies suggest that the dream-work is simply a translation, representing what a person thinks while asleep. An unanswered question was the exact nature of the relationship between spontaneous and hypnotic dreams, and whether censorship could be expected to manifest itself in the latter.[2]

Hypnosis provides a unique opportunity of studying the dynamic interaction involved in the acquisition and modification of the significance of signs and symbols, and a third study focused attention on the mode of symbolic transformation per se.

Four hospitalized, neurotic patients were again trained to produce hypnotic dreams, a procedure providing the opportunity to observe the transformation of a suggested content into its symbolic equivalent. An important innovation was the training of subjects to project *static* symbolic images on an imagined movie screen, such that a single symbol would depict a suggested content. Freud recognized that dream symbols are typically overde-

[2] Authorities are not agreed as to the exact relationship between hypnotic and spontaneous night dreams. M. Brenman (1949) states, "It is curious that investigators appear to have taken it for granted that the hypnotic suggestion to 'dream' issues in a dream." She argues that hypnotic dreams are relatively oversimplified, less influenced by unconscious thought processes, and are basically motivated by the desire to preserve the relationship with the hypnotist rather than preservation of sleep. However, this argument is greatly weakened by her admission that spontaneous night dreams are by no means homogeneous in their expressive form and, like the hypnotically induced dream, may range from an embellished reminiscence to a highly elaborated, symbolized product. In contrast, M. Mazer (1951) states that a dream should be defined by the nature of the production, not by the circumstances of its occurrence, and that the hypnotic dream possesses all of the distortions characteristic of the regular night dream. It seems agreed that the hypnotically induced dream varies greatly, but that a general, unstructured posthypnotic suggestion to be carried out during regular sleep results in a product very similar to a spontaneous night dream. Present experiments are based on the assumption that hypnotic and spontaneous dreams are sufficiently similar in the employment of symbolism to allow cross-generalization.

termined, and this mechanism of condensation (in combination with displacement) was accorded primary responsibility for the unintelligibility of dreams. It is also a factor which greatly complicates precise semantic measurement. The present approach was an attempt to partially control the effect of condensation while studying displacement or symbolization. In addition, suggestions were restricted to the symbolization of simple, concrete sexual anatomy and activities. Abstract latent content is often difficult to rate against a denotative differential (just as a connotative differential was not applicable to many varieties of concrete manifest content). It was hoped to tailor both content levels for use with the denotative differential. This emphasis on sexual content was consistent with the psychoanalytic penchant for assigning sexual significance to dream symbols.[3]

Sometimes subjects responded with a single symbolization; they also responded with series of symbols, each representing the suggested content. For instance, one female subject was unhappily married and possessed an intense fear, dislike, and envy of men. When asked to symbolize the male organ, she perceived in rapid succession: "A knife, a bull with tremendous horns, an enema bulb." Her hypnotic associations revealed that she thought of men as aggressively assaulting women. She also produced a vivid memory of impotent rage toward her mother who frequently "violated me" with enemas as a child. Her symbolizations of the female organ were also revealing of highly personal attitudes: "An outhouse, a pedestrian traffic-tunnel (where men urinate), a door on which hung a sign 'No Peddlers or Agents,' and a new green car parked beside a pile of breadcrusts." The last represented her envy of male prerogatives. This approach allowed objective measurement and identification of the elements

[3] A characteristic suggestion given subjects was as follows: "In a moment you will fall deeply asleep. When you do, a dream will form. You will find yourself seated in a movie theater looking at a blank screen. You will then clearly see (a suggested sexual content) followed immediately by a second picture or series of pictures which represent or stand for the same thing, just as you might have experienced it in a dream."

of meaning common to a variety of symbolizations of a single latent content.

The possible methodological variations provided by hypnosis in the study of the symbolic process in action are practically unlimited, and several additional approaches are suggested in the following examples. Subjects were instructed to project a series of static symbols, each of which would become increasingly transparent in meaning until the latent content was directly represented (a desymbolizing process). For example, when an unmarried female subject was given a suggestion to symbolize the male genitalia, she responded: "I see a couple of small peanuts. They are moving about, they won't stand still. Now they have spots like potatoes. Sprouts are growing out of the spots — they are changing, curving. It looks like a unicorn with a horn on its nose. I just see the head. There are circular lines around the horn. The head is changing again, into a sac — it is wrinkled. Oh! testicles and penis!"

A more detailed experiment with the same subject will demonstrate the potentialities inherent in another variation, that of directly suggesting the symbols a subject should use to depict a specified content.

1) The subject rated three sexual concepts on the differential, PENIS, VAGINA, INTERCOURSE, interspersed among a dozen irrelevant (nonsexual) concepts. Hypnosis was then induced and she was instructed to fall deeply asleep and to have a dream of being seated in a movie theater looking at a blank screen. She was instructed to perceive the male sex organ on the screen, to be followed immediately by a second picture which represented or stood for the same thing, "just as you might experience it in your dreams."

2) The patient signaled the beginning and termination of a dream. Still under hypnosis she reported having seen "a man with no clothes on — the lower part of his body. *It* looked big and hard and bony. It gave me a funny feeling in my stomach." She reported that this image was then replaced by a "necktie with a

tight knot in the end of it." The patient was told that when she awakened she would be amnesic for this episode until a given signal, whereupon she would remember *only* the necktie (not its covert meaning).

3) The patient awoke, smiled, and apologized, saying that she must have dozed off. Questioning elicited no apparent memory for what had transpired. She was then asked to rate the general concept NECKTIE on the differential. Next she was asked her associations to the concept. "An article of men's wearing apparel. I think of them as being attractive. They are so versatile and come in so many different shapes, colors, sizes, and designs. I also think of them as reflecting the personalities of the men who wear them."

4) At the prearranged signal she instantly and with seeming surprise recalled the necktie she perceived on the screen (but not its association with the male organ). She was asked to visualize the scene as vividly as possible, and then to rate this specific necktie on the differential (refer to Fig. 1).[4]

5) The patient entered a second hypnotic trance, and was again told to perceive the movie screen and upon it the now familiar necktie, but that this time the necktie would depict the female genitalia.[5] She was again requested to be amnesic for the suggestion. Upon indication that the "dream" had ceased, she awoke and stated that she had again seen the necktie but that this time it was a "red necktie, just about the reddest necktie you can

---

[4] The distance measure developed by Osgood and Suci (1952) is a statistical procedure particularly applicable to differential measurements. This method takes into account both the absolute discrepancy between sets of measurements and their profile similarity. The basis for the method is the generalized distance formula, $D = \sqrt{d^2}$. The operation for finding the semantic distance (D) between any two concepts is extremely simple; one sums the squared differences for a pair of variables (concepts) and takes the square root of the total. When identical sets of scales are employed in the judgment of different concepts, this method makes it possible to compare various differentiations of the same concept at various times or under various conditions in terms of their over-all meaningful similarity.

[5] Another test of a prevalent psychoanalytic belief suggests itself here. To paraphrase Jones (1950, p. 98), an individual is free to choose his dream symbols or to make new ones; what he cannot do is to give a regular (universal) symbol a different meaning.

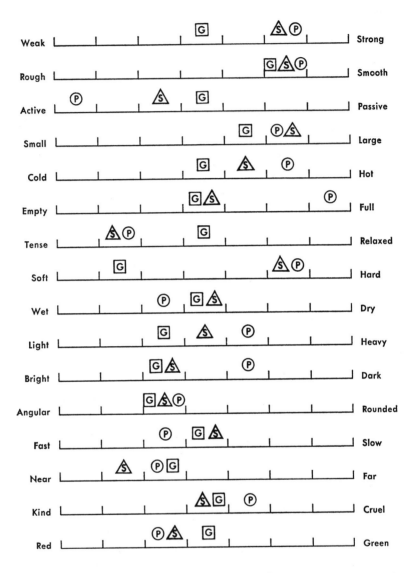

FIG. 1. Comparison of three concepts: PENIS ⓟ, rated prior to experiment; NECKTIE ⑤, as an unconscious symbol for penis, rated in dream context; NECKTIE Ⓖ, general or nonsymbol, rated later out of the dream context. Quantitative relationships (D statistic): penis vs. necktie-nonsymbol = 7.68; penis vs. necktie-symbol = 4.80; necktie-nonsymbol vs. necktie-symbol = 5.48 (the smaller the number, the closer the relationship).

imagine; it had a crease down the center of it and seemed quite curved."

6) She rated this new necktie on the differential. Asked to associate to the new tie, she replied, "The red makes me think of something that is very bright and active, something which is very stimulating, it is definitely more feminine than most colors that men will wear" (refer to Fig. 2).

7) The subject was placed in a third hypnotic state and was instructed that this time she would briefly witness herself having intercourse, and that this scene would then be replaced by another picture representing the same thing to her; she was told to remember only the latter scene.

After signaling completion of the dream, the subject reported that she had seen "a hotdog between two slices of bun. It was an extremely large hotdog, pointing straight upwards, and also there was a large slice of onion between it and the bun." She was instructed to be amnesic for the entire experience.

8) Upon awakening the subject was asked to rate HOTDOG on the differential. By a prearranged signal she next remembered the hotdog seen on the screen (but not the immediately preceding scene or latent content) and was asked to rate it.

9) The patient was returned to a hypnotic state and was asked to associate to each of the symbols she had used and to attempt an interpretation of their meaning.

First necktie: "As I said before, an article of men's clothing, something intimately related to a man, something definitely masculine. The straightness of it makes me think maybe it is starched or stiff. The knot in the end looks like, well, like a man's organ."

Second necktie: "That reminds me of a man's organ, too, but it's different somehow. The curve reminds me of the curve of a woman's body. The red makes me think of something that is very much alive; it makes me think of the vagina. I connect the idea of redness with the act of menstruation. I feel afraid of the penis though I know it would not really hurt me, but I am

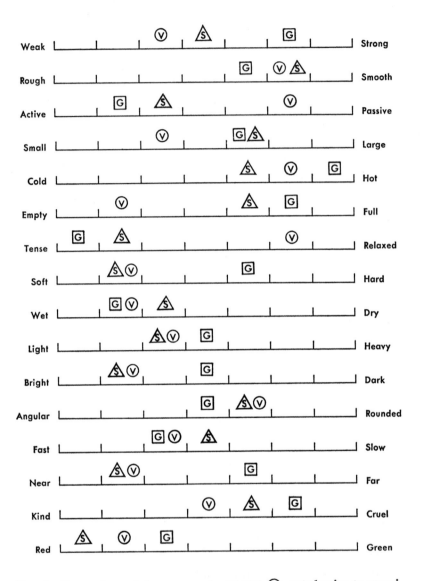

FIG. 2. Comparison of three concepts: VAGINA Ⓥ, rated prior to experiment; NECKTIE △ₛ, a male symbol which subject was required to use as a female symbol, rated in the dream context; NECKTIE Ⓖ, nonsymbol, rated out of the dream context. Quantitative relationships: vagina vs. necktie–female symbol = 7.28; vagina vs. penis = 11.22; intercourse vs. necktie–female symbol = 6.56; vagina vs. necktie-nonsymbol = 6.40; intercourse vs. necktie-nonsymbol = 7.81.

afraid it would make me pregnant. The vagina is not pregnant when it menstruates. The crease down the front of the tie is actually the opening of the woman's organ, and the curve is the shape of the vagina, too. Actually, this necktie is both male and female, but the female seems to predominate. The first necktie was only the penis. Both of them are stimulating, but the second is more so. It sort of makes me think of a penis being in a vagina, that is, of sexual intercourse."

Hotdog: "Well, the hotdog is the penis, too. It is very pointed and it is slanted — it is slanting away from me. This causes the thought that I mustn't touch it because it would make me pregnant. The bun is the vagina, and the fact that it is holding the wiener indicates that sexual intercourse is taking place. The whiteness of the onion indicates purity to me — the need to avoid having intercourse so that pregnancy will not occur. It, and the slant of the hotdog, and the redness of the necktie all represent the same thing — the need to avoid sexual contact."

10) The patient was obviously rather distressed at this point and was reluctant to talk further about her feelings. She responded that the hotdog had brought up a "forgotten" subject to her, "something that I had put out of my mind and refused to even think about anymore." She then related that six months previously she had gone on a picnic with her boyfriend and they had experienced intercourse for the first time. She spontaneously recalled a specific memory of lying wrapped in the blanket with him after having completed the act, glancing up over his shoulder, and seeing a half-eaten, shriveled hotdog. She laughed and commented that it looked like his "hotdog." Thus, the choice of the symbol produced in the experimental situation was apparently determined by this repressed but dynamically active experience. She further volunteered that later she had experienced several nightmares in which she was choking on a hotdog, and that in the past six months for reasons until now unknown to her, hotdogs had become completely unappetizing.

It is of considerable interest to note that the subject is not merely a symbolizing automaton but responds with symbolic productions which graphically depict personal needs and problems. Rich potentialities for the clinical employment of this technique as a projective method for personality exploration have been suggested (Watkins, 1956). Here the suggestion activated a very real conflict situation for the subject, reflecting both sensitivity of the method and the precautions that must be observed in its experimental application.

The remainder of this chapter will deal with one specific application of the demonstrated methods, the study of the process of cognitive interaction involved in meaning formation and change which Osgood refers to as the principle of congruity (Osgood et al., 1957, p. 200). Briefly, this principle states that whenever two signs having different meanings (different mediation processes and different profiles against the semantic differential) are related, the meaning of each shifts toward agreement with the other, the magnitude of the shift being *inversely proportional to the intensity* (degree of polarization, as reflected on the differential) of the interacting reactions. Two signs are said to be congruent to the extent that their mediating reactions are equally intense, either in the same (compatible) direction or in the opposite direction. Results obtained in the reported investigations suggest several features concerning the process of dream symbol acquisition and modification.

1) At the moment of symbol selection a situation exists in which the latent impulse "scans" a pool of potential symbols which share one or more physionomic qualities with the content to be represented (e.g., the similarity in shape between hotdog and penis). Logically, the analogy may be quite tenuous, of course. Differences are largely disregarded, with two important exceptions: (a) Each dream has a general theme or setting (e.g., psychotherapy = a dangerous ocean voyage) determined by the predominant affect and the selection of one or two key symbols. The remaining symbols will tend to be consistent (e.g., gangplank = resistance, ship captain = therapist, cabin = sleep,

etc.). This gives the dream its theatrical quality. (b) The *prein-teraction* location of the potential symbol in relation to the latent content cannot be highly incongruent with respect to the emotional aspects of meaning. This would appear to account for seeming preference for symbols which, in their own right (independent of the dream context), are often innocuous or affectively neutral.

2) The fact that the latent content has, typically, powerful associated affective and cognitive processes, which in combination with the affectively neutral (or possibly congruent) potential symbol, determines the flow of significance from the primary sign (A) to the secondary idea or symbol (B). These observations are completely predictable from the principle of congruity. The more polarized one sign is, relative to the other, the less change it undergoes. Where one member of an assertion is neutral, *all* the shift in meaning is concentrated on this concept.

3) Insofar as B receives its meaning from identification with A, it functions as its symbolic equivalent. In the dream a momentary situation obtains in which the interaction is maximized; that is, the meaning of each sign is shifted totally to the point of mutual congruence. At this moment the dreamer is completely credulous: he accepts the symbol as reality. However, the tendency is, after such cognitive interaction, for the meanings of related signs to "bounce" back to their original locus, and the whole phenomenon has a mercurial quality which defies direct measurement, although the employment of hypnotic techniques allows almost immediate access to and reproducibility of this symbol-making process. When the dreamer awakens, there will be a reduction in the congruity effect both as a function of time and an altered state of consciousness (the semantic distance between latent and manifest content increases to the point where dream symbols become largely unintelligible).

It should be noted that when the affect associated with the primary idea is too intense (as in the last case example), an individual continues to experience a continuing, disturbing, logically

incomprehensible identity of signs (hotdogs = intercourse) resulting in a phobic reaction, or in the extreme case, a psychotic
delusion or hallucination.

SUMMARY

Several forms of Osgood's semantic differential were employed
in the study of spontaneous and hypnotically induced dreams.
While the use of hypnosis to investigate symbolization is not
original with these studies, the feasibility of objectification of this
elusive psychological phenomenon has been demonstrated, including a step toward identification of the psychological laws underlying the acquisition and modification of sign significance. The
primary intent of the chapter is to stimulate and provoke experimentation in an important area of human behavior long resistant
(resisted) to scientific investigation.

THREE

The Hypnotic Interpretation of Dreams: A Clinical Experiment

INTRODUCTION

This is a highly elaborated case study of the ability of a single patient-subject to use hypnosis in the interpretation of his own spontaneous nocturnal dreams, a procedure which led to the successful termination of treatment in a relatively brief period of time. This case was the introduction to the author of the possibilities in the use of hypnosis for the exploration of unconsciously produced symbolism.[1] The patient-subject for this clinical experiment was a 28-year-old white male, married and employed as an

[1] Let us briefly trace the development of how the author selected this dissertation topic. In attempting to formulate hypotheses on the use of hypnosis in studying dreams, he was highly influenced by the then recent book of David Rapaport's, *The Organization and Pathology of Thought* (1951). It contained dozens of untranslated European papers related to thought disorganization and Rapaport provided a very scholarly critique of them. One section contained papers by Schroetter, Roffenstein, and Nachmansohn, the three Viennese physicians who had performed studies using hypnosis to investigate dreams during the period 1910–25. The author was intrigued with the discussion and the relative paucity of further studies on the subject matter.

The author began testing his patients to determine whether any of them had a facility for dealing with dreams under hypnosis — and he established that some of his patients did exhibit such an aptitude, even under his crude attempts with hypnosis. He also quickly learned that no technique provided him with such singular insight into the lives and perceptions of his patients or held such a potential for treatment. Paradoxically, he had also developed many scientific reservations about the way that psychoanalysts conducted dream interpretation with their patients.

inventory stock clerk. His first hospitalization had occurred 11
years earlier, when as a military noncombatant overseas, he made
a suicidal gesture. A depressive reaction failed to respond to treatment, and he was eventually given a medical discharge. Upon
entry into the current treatment program he suffered multiple somatic complaints.

The patient became acutely aware of his own unhappiness at a
young age. In an autobiographical sketch written at age 18, he acknowledged that his family made him nervous because of their
constant bickering. "It seemed as if we were always fighting
about something and nothing that I did ever pleased them." Even
then he was concerned about his physical condition: "My health
was always bad — colds, stomach upsets — and I never seemed
to have much pep." He also admitted to episodes of depression in
early youth. His general attitude toward people is contained in
the statement, "I try to stay away from them, they make me
sick." The family physician characterized the patient as always
having been "lean, sluggish, asthenic, emotionally unstable . . .
a handicapped person . . . his trouble may be due to glands."

Following his military discharge the patient returned home
and resumed a familiar role of subjugation to the father. The patient wanted to attend dramatic school but feared his father's dis-
pleasure and allowed himself instead to be coerced into accoun-
tancy training. However, a recurrence of ill health soon forced
him to drop from school. Shortly thereafter he left for California
to recover his health, and by this act, for the first time in his life
directly disobeyed his father. One month's vacation was protracted into eight. Freed from parental prohibitions and restraints,
the patient rejected all responsibility, dated frequently and pro-
miscuously, and drank excessively. This period of abandon finally
terminated when the father suffered a debilitating heart attack
which necessitated the patient's return.

At home again the patient got a job and within a few months,
married. Subsequent marital discord brought about an exacerba-
tion of the patient's symptoms and was the acknowledged source

of his motivation in seeking therapy. The wife was extremely immature and, like the patient, was engaged in a dependency struggle with her own parents. Each partner experienced the dependency conflict of the other as a source of personal threat and reacted accordingly. At the time of entry into therapy the marriage held few satisfactions for either and the relationship had disintegrated to the point where communication was restricted to the hostile and mundane.

Despite a superior intellectual endowment (I.Q.=121), the patient impressed the therapist initially with his psychological naiveté. He exhibited minimal insight into the basis of his difficulties and a proneness to attribute them exclusively to an organic etiology. On the positive side, the patient appeared genuinely motivated and was able to interact effectively despite his anxiety. A good rapport was soon established. The patient was seen for a total of 48 sessions (which is perhaps at the upper boundary of what can be labeled "brief psychotherapy"). There was a perceptible pattern common to the majority of sessions, determined by the patient's ability to produce and interpret clinically rich and significant dreams. Associations obtained in reference to these dreams usually led directly to a discussion of important current problems. In this manner dreams became the focal point of most sessions, from which subsequent topics of discussion naturally ensued.

As indicated, the role of the therapist during much of therapy was predominantly supportive and nondirective, the patient being encouraged to initiate and pursue topics which he felt to be important. A cardinal manifestation of the transference relationship was the patient's insistence, in effect, on conducting his own therapy, beginning with the second session when he assumed the therapist's desk chair, next took over induction and then the termination of the hypnotic state, and finally produced and translated his own dreams. This dynamic, obviously related to a need to achieve independence from his domineering father was never challenged.

ILLUSTRATIVE DREAM PRODUCTIONS AND INTERPRETATIONS

Limitation of space prohibits reproduction of all 76 dreams (58 of sufficient length to merit analysis), or the interpretations, waking and hypnotic, given them by the patient during the course of treatment. Four episodes have been chosen as representative of the employment of this approach in the conduct of psychotherapy. It should be re-emphasized that the patient's proficiency in producing meaningful associations to his dreams in hypnosis allowed complete avoidance of arbitrary therapist-imposed interpretations. Nor were special techniques required in order to integrate the insights achieved in hypnosis, since during the subsequent discussion in each session, the patient exhibited a spontaneous transition to a fully functioning, awake state. That is to say, whereas initially a formal induction procedure was necessary, with practice the subject learned to induce and to terminate hypnosis himself, thus further promoting the nondirective character of the proceedings.

Most of the initial session was spent by the patient in recitation of the events immediately preceding the request for treatment. Despite the reiteration that his difficulties were purely organic in basis, the patient did admit that this construction had been challenged by repeated physical examinations which produced negative results. By the conclusion of the hour the patient appeared relatively at ease. Upon departure he was told that he might bring to the next session any dreams he had in the intervening period. The very first dream of the patient appears in Chapter Two, pp. 16–18.

Session X

Dream. He was in the recreation hall of his former university in company with two other fellows. The three of them were going to play bridge or cards. They decided there was not room enough and one of the others said that he knew a place to play. The others left the room while the patient gathered up the cards, paper, and pencil and followed. He found himself alone and at the head of a long flight of stairs. When he reached the bottom he found two archways, one right and one left. The one to the right had a bitch lying in the doorway nursing her puppies. The patient went left and entered a hallway filled with busy workmen hammering and sawing. He next entered a large room which was empty except for a small pickup truck parked in the center. He found that his sport clothes had changed to work clothes in the meantime. He then perceived his friend coming down a flight of stairs from an office. His friend stated, "We had better hurry or we'll be late." He felt somewhat angry and thought "Why the hell did he lead me down here to work?"

Interpretation. There were no meaningful awake associations; an understanding of the dream was revealed by the patient's associations in hypnosis. In one respect it was a transference dream, i.e., it reflected the patient's attitudes toward therapy and the therapist. Briefly, the patient came into therapy and found it interesting and stimulating intellectually (à la *university*). He made progress and it was fairly satisfying. Then he suddenly found himself blocked, frustrated, and unable to continue his progress. On the upper or conscious level, he gets along fairly well (therapy is like a "game of chance"). But once he passes beneath the surface via hypnosis (*stairs*), he found the going difficult. The *workmen* represent his defenses and they are busy altering and erecting barriers to free communication in therapy. He finds that he is angry with the therapist (*friend*) for not having given him adequate warning of the difficulties he would encounter; he feels indignant that the "fun" has turned into work. "I was sailing along and all of a sudden it seemed to me to be hard work. I now realize that it takes work both to attain and maintain progress. It is like walking on an icy street; there is always the danger of slipping and falling back again." [2]

[2] Every patient comes into treatment asking the therapist to relieve him of anxiety; he doesn't realize how difficult psychotherapy will soon become. It eventually dawns upon the patient as it did in this case, after nine sessions, that a great deal of "hard work" is called for. At this point, he becomes ambivalent and resistant. This is correct regardless of the form of treatment, but it is especially true in hypnotic treatment because of the connotations of a magical cure.

The dream also depicts an ambivalent feeling towards his wife. The *bitch nursing pups* signifies a barrier that has long existed between the patient and his wife, namely, her desire to have a baby as opposed to his economic fears. This dream followed an evening in which the patient was persuaded by his wife that they should at last have a baby and they had intercourse that night without contraception. However, the patient is still clearly ambivalent; in fact, in the dream he seemingly rejects the idea. The archway to the right signifies the entrance way to his wife, and the doorway to the left is filled with workmen erecting obstacles to the therapy relationship. The *pickup truck* represents the patient's desire to escape from the responsibility of both marriage and psychotherapy, allowing him to regress into his neurosis.

Session XXII

The patient reported "a terrible week." His cold had continued and he had developed "piles" for the first time in his life. "A couple of times I felt like just jumping out of the window." He had first suffered diarrhea, followed by pain during elimination. He related an extremely terrifying nightmare which had awakened him last night.

There were two identical log cabins facing each other, connected by two sets of stairways which met at the bottom. In the cabins were rival factions composed of several individuals. The leader of the group to which the patient and his wife belonged left and went next door, seemingly in search of the opposing leader. He stormed about the room destroying furniture, and then seized the terrified wife of the absent leader, lifted her, broke her back over his knee, and threw her out the window. He then returned to the first cabin and retired to a bedroom. The individuals in this cabin (including the patient and his wife) were filled with anxious anticipation. The patient reassured his wife that he had rigged an alarm which would tell them if anyone opened the door and that in any event she would be protected. Suddenly the door literally splintered and in the doorway stood a huge monster. Without a word, he strode into the room and implanted an axe in the chest of the cabin leader's wife. She was surprised and horrified and in terrible pain sank into a chair with her hand over the wound. The giant jerked out the axe and disappeared into the bedroom. Then came a scream and the sound of an axe chopping into flesh. The patient recalled feeling nauseated and disgusted. He grabbed a poker from the fireplace with the idea that if he was attacked, he would stab the monster in the eyes and blind him. He awoke feeling very ill.

The patient by this time had gained proficiency in hypnosis and it was suggested to him that the dream was incomplete. Under hypnosis the original dream was revivified and then was continued past the point of original termination with the following results:

The monster returned to the room and the patient attacked him with the prongs and succeeded in ripping him open. To the patient's astonishment the monster was filled with sawdust. "He was like a robot, controlled by somebody else, but there were no real parts." The more the patient ripped, the more the monster disintegrated into a pile of sawdust. The patient then sat down in amazement and just stared at it.

According to the patient's hypnotically induced associations (he blocked completely in the waking state), this was the meaning of the dream:

The *monster* represents the tremendous store of hate which the patient has long accumulated toward his father, brother, and wife, powerful emotions which he had somehow forced himself to control. However, these sessions have allowed him to examine and analyze his feelings, thus threatening his tenuous controls. The hypnotically stimulated sequel seemed to depict an attempt at denial of the validity of these hostile feelings and recognition that much of his hatred is senseless, that is, attributed to his own behavior.

The monster represents "a hate grown to monstrous proportions" but it also represents the hate evidenced by his brother and father as well, especially the brother. The patient feels that it is evil to hate and that a person who hates without basis is evil. "Maybe I've thought all along that I had a basis for my hate but actually I haven't. Perhaps 'restriction' is the cause, that is, I've been forced to withhold my emotions so long that they have grown into hatred."

The woman murdered by the monster represents both the wife and the mother, and the patient felt disgust with himself for his brutality. He recalled with remorse the occasions when his wife had tried to communicate with him. "I've come to realize that maybe she has felt the same way that I did and wasn't able to express her feelings either. The whole dream seems to represent the senselessness of my bad feelings. If you tear them apart, then there is no reason for them."

The two log cabins represent the idea that there are two sides to everything, that two individuals can view the same situation and come out with identical emotions but opposed attitudes. "There can be two different points of view but actually they are the same. In my relations with my parents and my wife, it would help if I could see things from their points of view and how they feel about it." [3]

This led to a discussion of his inability to express his emotions. "I feel them and want to express them but I am paralyzed." He drew the analogy of the prisoner who bore a ball and chain so long that even after he was freed, he was unable to walk without dragging a foot; i.e., even though the patient can now see the virtue of expressing his feelings, suppression has been so ingrained that he cannot do so even though he wishes it.

Space permits only a cursory presentation of the genetics and dynamic content elicited in treatment. The patient came from a semiorthodox Jewish home. His father was a strict disciplinarian, domineering, self-aggrandizing, impatient, captious, and intolerant of any challenge to his absolute authority. He had little time for the family members, preferring solitary pursuits such as tinkering with his car. In contrast, the mother was meek, hard-

---

[3] Every single symbol has significance, is woven into a fabric of the dream, and contributes to the over-all meaning. Take any symbol or two and it rapidly expands into several paragraphs of logical, waking meaning for the dreamer. This is an additional illustration that the dream is a greatly condensed form of language. A dream symbol really is worth a thousand words!

working, and long-suffering. Although she was for the patient the preferred parent, her love and attention were quite apparently insufficient to generate feelings of personal worth and security in him. Both mother and patient reacted to the father with complete submissiveness, the latter tending to suppress, repress, and deny intense feelings of resentment. In early adolescence the patient became increasingly withdrawn and found himself preoccupied with thoughts of retaliation and eventual emancipation for his mother and himself. His life motif became, "Do unto others as others have done unto you."

The family constellation was completed by a younger brother. In contrast to the patient who was asthenic in build and delicate in health, the brother was a robust physical specimen who had always bullied the patient. Possessed of an aggressive temperament, he rebelled against the father, and their relationship was punctuated with frequent violent quarrels. The brother's behavior was experienced by the patient as a threat since it activated his own "death wishes" toward the older man. Because the brother was an agitator and dissenter, it was incomprehensible to the patient that both parents seemed to prefer the former.

Session XXXIX

The patient stated that on Saturday evening he had an "attack of nerves," meaning stomach pains and cramps, chills, and diarrhea (a recurrence of the somatic difficulties had markedly decreased in recent sessions). The patient reported that he and his wife had visited friends and he had eaten food which had not agreed with him. In characteristic fashion, he could see no other possible cause for his digestive upset. He vaguely referred to office pressures as a possible source of tension: "I've been feeling that perhaps I had bitten off more than I could chew."

The patient entered hypnosis and was told that he would experience a spontaneous flow of memories intimately related to his digestive upset. He immediately perceived four scenes from the previous Saturday which constituted a chronology of disturbing events. These events were taken up in detail, each being reinstated in turn through vivification and time regression.[4]

1) The patient's wife was to meet him so he could give her a driving lesson. The patient completes work at 11:15 and begins waiting for his wife. At 11:45 he calls home but no one is there. At 12:05 he becomes so angry that he starts to leave, at which time she finally calls. The patient describes himself as extremely angry and irritated. He recalls thinking: "Why the hell can't she be more considerate of me? She sleeps all morning, can't she get up early just once? She just doesn't care! The same thing happened last week. She said that she had been talking on the phone to her girl friend and couldn't get away. What's more important, talking to her girl friend or keeping me waiting?" The patient feels 'hate' over this inconsiderate action. He also feels that the fellows in the office are laughing at him because of the way his wife treats him. He describes his stomach as "nervous, it's turning and twisting," an action which began when he started waiting for his wife.

2) "We are at the table. Mother has everything that I don't like." He persuades her to scramble him some eggs but she refuses to fry onions with them because she doesn't have the time. He feels angry and aggravated. "She knew I was coming but she didn't think enough of me to have the food that I liked. It's an insult — her lack of consideration." Patient becomes aware that his stomach is "churning harder" now. "If I were to let loose I would really tell them off. But I won't because I would just make enemies."

3) The patient and his father are working on the patient's car. The father, a skilled mechanic, is doing most of the work. One of the neighbors comes to watch and the father apologizes for his son's lack of mechanical ability. This makes the patient ex-

---

[4] These are highly important hypnotic techniques. It is possible to regress patients through hypnotic intensification of emotion. The subject may be told that upon signal from the hypnotherapist, whatever emotion that he is feeling will grow stronger and stronger with every second, until he experiences it completely. He may then spontaneously or on cue regress to another period, earlier in his life, when he felt exactly the same way.

tremely angry. "I wanted to tell him that he couldn't have done it alone. I was mad because he insists on treating me like a baby. So I'm not a mechanic, that is no reason to treat me as if I were nothing! I feel as if I would really like to bust him one, to hit him and to knock him down. There is a grinding in my stomach. My hate is something hard and deeply imbedded."

4) It is now evening and the patient and his wife are at their friends' home. They, too, have food for supper which the patient knows he should not eat. Finally he feels that he can't "stomach" this lack of consideration any longer and eats some corned beef though he knows it will not agree with him. After supper they play cards and he mentions to his wife that tomorrow he will take the car back to his father's for more work. She then casually informs him that this will be impossible because she has invited her parents for supper and he has to transport them. This infuriates the patient but he gives no overt expression because he fears precipitating an argument. "I feel that I am going to burst, that I'm filled to the breaking point with hate and anger. My stomach is really grinding and twisting now." An hour later the patient, having continued to smoulder, suddenly develops a full-blown digestive upset.

At this juncture the patient spontaneously recalled a dream which had occurred Saturday night.

Patient was standing in the street beside a car. Suddenly two huge people appeared, one on the left and one on the right. They started shooting at each other. Patient then found a gun in his hand, a very small, tiny gun. He took turns shooting at each of the big people but his shots were quite ineffective. Finally he was out of bullets and he said to one of the big people, "Now you can shoot me." This person appeared to be a Negro. Suddenly there was another gun on the seat of the car. This one was much larger and more effective looking than the last. The patient no longer felt frustrated and was just about to shoot with it when he awakened.

Hypnotic associations. "This is similar to the last few dreams I've reported in here. It symbolizes the hate which is coming out of me."

Person on the right: "He is on the defensive, he isn't taking too much action. He is rather tall and thin. He seems to shirk. He reminds me of myself, the way I am."

Person on the left: "Big, heavy set, dark-skinned, full-faced, he has a husky build, the way I would like to be built. He's aggressive but calm and intent, he can express emotion but has control of it. Possibly it's the way that I appear to others, though I know it is really just a facade. He is tan, brown, maybe it's egotistical but I like to have people tell me how good I look. Someone who is big, dark, strong and self-sufficient. The two people seem to represent me fighting with myself. The person on the left in some ways reminds me of my brother."

Car: "A means of escape."

The new gun: "The therapy situation and you."

First gun: "My silence and keeping things to myself — which doesn't get me anyplace."

Second gun: "Being able to talk and to get things off my chest."

Waking association. The patient recalled walking through the Merchandise Mart at noon and looking at a gun collection. He told a friend that he thought he should get one for the house — for protection. "But I know that I lied. I'd just like to blow some people's heads off — my father, a couple of my bosses, yes, even my wife!" Patient then recalled that he must have been ill prior to supper on Saturday night because upon arriving he had asked for some aspirin.

The remainder of the time was spent in discussion of the elicited material. At the end of the hour the patient expressed amazement that he had previously been unable to perceive the causal relationship between his emotional upset and the digestive disturbances which had followed.

Session XLIII

The patient characterized this as another miserable week.

Dream. Patient, wife, and a second man went to a concert, where they were seated on the left side of the balcony. His wife was looking at the program and wished they would change it for another. The music began and on stage below a woman began singing. Beside her was a man who suddenly slipped out a dagger. Both the patient and the man with him recognized immediately that this was not part of the act and the second man said, "We have to do something quick," whereupon the patient grabbed a nearby rope or sash and swung down from the balcony and swept over the stage. As he went by he struck the man with the knife and then swung up to a platform on the other side of the auditorium. While lying there he suddenly perceived that there was blood dripping onto the stage and that it was his. As he watched he saw the man below engage in combat with a man and a woman. Suddenly the man with the knife broke loose and plunged the weapon into the throat of the woman. She fell with the knife sticking in her throat and yelling for help. The second man then chased the killer into the wings. The patient was horrified by the whole event. He also remembered thinking about his wound, "No, this can't happen to me, it isn't true."

The patient was instructed to enter hypnosis and to re-experience the dream in all of its original intensity. He recalled his wife's first words as "No, I don't want that one now, make that one last and make the other next." He also added that the man who fought with the killer was the same one who was in the balcony with him but is still unable to identify him.

Hypnotic associations. It became immediately clear to the patient that the man and the woman on the stage represented his parents and the scene depicted "all the years that I can remember my father hurting my mother." He then had a spontaneous memory of the possible instigating factor of the dream: "Ellen told me Sunday that she had talked to Mother when we were there for dinner and that Mother had told her that a year after she married Dad, she became pregnant but obtained an abortion because she did not feel that she could properly take care of both children at that time." Patient says his reaction was a mixture of sorrow and gratitude: sorrow that she had to lose her child and gratitude that she should think enough of him to do such a thing. "I've always held the opinion that Dad didn't marry her because he loved her but so that he would have someone to take care of me."

He next recalled the many quarrels he had heard and seen them engage in as a child. The patient's reaction was one of extreme hate, a desire to do the father physical harm. He also described how lonely and lost he felt. "I wish that my mother wouldn't pay so much attention to the home and more to me."

Another scene then appeared. It was at the time of his engagement and his mother called him into the kitchen where she and the father were, to inform him that the father had decided that he wanted a divorce. "I was flabbergasted. All I remember is that I wanted to hurt him for what he was doing to Mother. I thought that the best way to hurt him was just not to show any interest, so I said, 'Well, he's old enough to know what he wants to do,' and turned and walked out. I felt that it was a good chance to take revenge on him. I didn't care what he did. I just felt 'Good riddance of bad rubbish.' Now I'll get an apartment and I'll take care of Mother. I felt stupefied by it all."

It was then suggested that the patient have a fantasy which would reveal the essential meaning of the dream. "I see Mother all worn and tired, and I see Dad standing over her like an overlord. I try to reach Mother but I can't save her. Something is holding me back. I don't know what it is." It was then suggested to the patient that he perceive a word which would represent this obstacle. He clearly saw "lack of affection." "Because they never showed any affection to me now I can't show them any affection. I feel it but I can't display it. Also, I've always been afraid of my father and that kept me from showing how I felt too. And the hate which I held for him — that was always in the way. I could never talk to either of them and so after a while I just gave up trying — whatever I felt I just kept inside. I still feel that I am unable to save Mother, but I also feel now that I'll get there in time, even though she must take punishment a little longer."

The patient was now able to make this interpretation of his dream: the *two men in the balcony* represent the two sides of the patient. The *stranger* is that aspect of himself which he had been upon coming into therapy, "the reserved, cold side that wants to do something but doesn't know how." The actual self in the dream is "the man of action who isn't afraid to speak his mind and to do what he wants — the individual that I feel perhaps I can become." About the dream in general: "I was thinking this week about Mother as you told me to do [an instruction from the previous session was to think of the role which the mother had played in his life, a subject which had been only lightly touched upon heretofore]. In the past I hadn't been able to see how I was acting, partly because I had always lived with myself, if you know what I mean. Now I'm beginning to see how I acted and reacted. All these feelings about Mother and Dad just seemed to come out during the week. I wondered if I couldn't make it easier for Mother by showing her more affection than I had. I felt so strongly the need to change, to be different, I couldn't show that affection if I continued to act as I had in the past."

Regarding his wife's short verbalization at the beginning of the dream, he now interpreted this to mean, "She isn't able to show her feelings for me yet, but later she will be able to." He stated the realization that part of her difficulty was due to his own un-responsiveness and part of the fact that she, too, had come from a family situation in which she had been trained to withhold her feelings. At this point the patient recognized the parallel processes at work in the father's relationship to the mother and his relationship to his wife. "Seemingly without realizing it, I've been treating her the same way Dad treated Mother." It was suggested that this become a topic for thought in the week ahead. With emphasis the patient stated, "I know now that I can change myself."

In reference to his expression at the conclusion of the dream, "This can't be true: everything that has come out here, all the things that I've learned about myself, my reaction is, *it can't be me!*" He also had an association to his work situation: "It can't be happening to me, that they won't let me go any further." Being in the balcony or on the platform and watching the scene below was to the patient "like watching the events of the past going before my eyes — it's representative of all the fights they've always had. I felt that the threat of divorce was akin to cutting out my mother's heart. Swinging down on the sash was like the brush-off which I gave my father in the kitchen — but without any effect."

Asked to tell how he now felt introspectively, the patient replied, "I feel all worked up — there is a gnawing in my stomach, and I feel like I've been crying. I'd like to tell Mother about all these things I've seen and undergone in here, but I don't know how she would react to it all." At the end of this time the patient was characteristically wide awake and the last 10 minutes were spent in working through this material on a purely conscious level.

In the final several sessions, effort was directed toward achieving an integration and synthesis of the therapeutic experience, again through the vehicle of the patient's interpretation of his own spontaneous night dreams. It was suggested there would spin before his eyes while hypnotized all the dreams he had experienced during therapy and that when the spinning stopped, he would re-experience one of the dreams which he had not interpreted and which he felt retrospectively was extremely important. Following this suggestion, he responded with dreams from several earlier sessions, supplying added interpretations or dealing with nuances of his interpretations.

In the final session, the patient was asked whether he had followed an instruction to think about therapy and the therapy relationship, but he responded that he was consciously aware of no particular feelings about the therapist. It was then suggested that he have a dream which would reveal his feelings. He responded with a short fantasy in which he was alternately striking the therapist in the face and offering him gifts. "On the one hand I want to hit you and on the other to repay you for all you have done to help me. I have mixed emotions. I want to hit you because you have made me look back on all these distasteful things, and on the other hand, I want to repay you for making me do so. I realize that only in this way can I lick the problem." He voiced surprise at his ambivalence, saying that he had been unaware of it. "Before it had just seemed to me that you were an instrument by which I might help myself, someone impersonal, and without too much feeling." Asked what seemed to prevent realization of true sentiments, he replied, "Fear that you would think I was trying to 'soft soap' you on the one hand, and fear that you would resent my hostility on the other." It was pointed out how this ambivalence and consequent blocking had been characteristic of him in all of his important relationships.

MODE OF SYMBOLIC REPRESENTATION

The themata of most reported dreams centered on the patient's current adjustment problems. Associated emotions were represented by personification, natural phenomena, objects, and activities. Hostile impulses, for example, were variously represented by an Indian, threatening weather conditions, and a ferocious bear. Anxiety was depicted by an attack of diarrhea, egocentric satisfactions by the eating of a candy bar, guarded emotions by money in a bank vault, emotional turmoil by turbulent water, a sense of well being by sunlight, and kissing as a prosaic symbolization for affection. Abstract ideas were also personified and transformed into concrete objects or activities. A clear example is a brief dream symbolizing the need to exclude bothersome sexual thoughts. The patient in his dream was watching a TV screen when there appeared a nude woman who stroked long pendulous breasts. His immediate reaction was, "Such scenes should be censored!" and the screen immediately went blank. Restrictions imposed by the pictorial mode of representation accounted for a type of imagery, namely, representations of multiplicity, which the patient found exceedingly difficult to translate in the waking state, although he could do so without hesitation in hypnosis. In one dream the divisions in a sidewalk referred to separate sessions of therapy, in another a line of girls represented different aspects of adjustment with the wife, and in a third dream 12 people represented the passage of time, i.e., "twelve hours in a day, twelve months in a year."

One virtue of the longitudinal study of a single subject was the opportunity to observe the consistency with which a recurring thema was represented by the same or closely related symbols. This finding supplements the observations of other investigators such as Mazer (1951), who employed a cross-sectional approach to the study of symbolization in the hypnotic dream and found the symbols used to depict a single thema were highly idiosyncratic, but the attitude displayed by individual subjects was quite consistent from one dream to the next. In this study, the symbols utilized were remarkably consistent, as were attitudes displayed. For instance, *water* appeared as a symbol in no less than 14 dreams, and each time it represented intense hostile impulses which threatened the patient's tenuous control. Repressive operations themselves were invariably represented by locked or guarded doors, rooms, private apartments, or containers. The symbol *cabin* was employed for this purpose in five different dreams and was identified in hypnosis as a "blockhouse, a place for guarded thoughts." Other specific symbols for defensive activities were walls, locker, fence, closet, armor, umbrella, rubbers, bank, condom, etc. The repressed hostile impulses were frequently personified by an *Indian* (a savage, cruel, warlike person whose behavior was justified by the treatment he received). In 13 dreams, hostile impulses were symbolized by a *weapon* such as a gun or a knife. In 12 dreams the patient depicted his neurotic adjustment as a *form of vehicle*, for example, convertible, Dodge truck, even a "soapbox" orange crate. In seven dreams psychotherapy was also represented by some *mode of transportation* (a means of getting from the old to the new), in six dreams as *fishing* or *boating*, and in five dreams it was portrayed as a *game of chance*.

The great majority of the patient's dreams were concerned

with current interpersonal difficulties. The patient was usually an active participant in a dream, though occasionally he was a detached observer. He cast himself in roles appropriate to the general context of the particular dream and was at different times a world traveler, hospital patient, fisherman, prison warden, missionary, high school student, bellhop, boxer, bank robber, and so forth. There were frequent multiple representations of self, or aspects of self, which the patient tended not to recognize in the waking state. Similarly, while representations of others were usually direct, the patient experienced difficulty in identifying the persons populating his dreams when they appeared in unconventional roles. Composite figures representing an identity of behavior or feeling between two or more persons were particularly confusing, as was the personification of an emotion or abstract idea. An absent person might also be alluded to by a personal, associated part, such as his hat or car, or sometimes an indirect verbal reference. The ease with which the subject understood these representations immediately when hypnotized was always impressive.

MANIFEST CONTENT ANALYSIS

The 58 dreams were "scored" on the following Hall–Van de Castle (1966) scales of manifest content: characters, objects, aggression, friendliness, sex, misfortunes, good fortune, success, failure, emotions, oral incorporation, castration anxiety, castration wish, and penis envy. The frequencies (usually expressed as proportions) for each of the categories were compared with the male norms given by Hall and Van de Castle. These norms are based on the analysis of 500 dreams reported by 100 male college students between the ages of 18 and 25. The following interpretations of the dreams were done by Calvin Hall and checked by his assistant, Vernon Nordby, without any knowledge of the analysis provided by the patient.

As is generally the case, a number of dreamer's proportions were virtually identical with the norms. There is a large universal factor in what people dream about. This factor tells about people in general but it does not reveal what is unique about an individual's personality. Consequently, attention will be focused on the deviations.

The outstanding deviations are the high incidence of aggression and the low incidence of friendliness and sex. There are no overt sex dreams at all, when according to the norms there should be six or seven. Aggression is high between the dreamer and all classes of characters: males, females, family members, known persons, strangers, and animals. The dreamer is more often the aggressor than the victim which is contrary to the norms. Friendliness is low with all classes of characters.

— With regard to characters, he dreams more about family members and strangers and less about friends and acquaintances than the norm group.

— He suffers more misfortunes and more failures in his dreams than the average male dreamer does. There is also more anxiety and penis envy.

— An interesting deviation appears in the object categories. There are many more implements in his dreams. In the Hall–Van de Castle system, implements are divided into three classes: tools, weapons, and recreational equipment. He is especially high in the tools and weapons categories.

The following inferences are drawn from the foregoing quantitative results. The dreamer lives in a world of enemies. There is no one he can trust and no one he can use as a shield against a hostile world. This would surely make him suspicious, insecure, and anxious. He has an array of negative feelings toward women. They are exploitative, castrating, rejecting, shady, and seductive. These attitudes toward women taken in conjunction with a high proportion of aggression with males means that he has no sanctuary. He is vulnerable from all sides. This is the pattern found in a study of mental patients (Hall, 1966).

The dreamer sees himself as being ineffectual. This ineffectualness is due to concern over masculinity, or more specifically, sexual potency. The high incidence of tools and weapons, anxiety, misfortune, failure, and penis envy suggests that he feels inadequately equipped as a male.

The dreamer is an enraged, ineffectual, anxious, impotent, castrated person. It would be assumed that he had a mother who rejected or castrated him, and a similar sort of wife. He is still enmeshed in the nexus of the family, and has not found his way to outside friendships. Aside from his family, he lives in a world of strangers.

It is unfortunate that Hall's method requires that the dreams be provided in a variable (randomized) sequence, which deprives them of any sequential analysis.

EXPERIMENTAL MEASURES OF THERAPEUTIC PROGRESS

Chronologically, the first half of treatment dealt primarily with an exploration of the patient's relationships with his father and brother. The patient experienced repeated cathartic release of long-suppressed resentments against all family members. The focus later shifted to the relationship with his wife and to a lesser extent with his mother. Emphasis throughout was upon the current problem situation, though an attempt was also made to develop a meaningful (recent) historical context. At the conclusion of treatment the patient was cognizant of many of the dynamic factors which had long determined his thoughts and actions, including an increased awareness of his own very sizable contribution to these difficulties, and it was felt by the therapist that sufficient momentum had been generated to insure continued progress.

Indications of improvement were numerous and varied. At the conclusion of treatment the patient seemed capable of actually dealing with problem situations on a more realistic level. Sporadic recurrences were later coincident with periods of acute stress, but at termination the patient was relatively symptom-free. The MMPI administered pre- and post-therapy reflects this alleviation of symptoms in the relative reduction on the "neurotic triad."

	Scales								
	Hs	D	Hy	Pd	Mf	Pa	Pt	Sc	Ma
First session:	67	65	69	57	57	65	56	52	58
Forty-eighth session:	49	59	49	54	55	59	54	63	58

In general, interpersonal relationships were no longer imbued with the same degree of threat and the patient became capable of relating without employment of numerous security measures. Similarly, the patient was better able to accept previously dissociated aspects of "self" with less dependence on mechanisms of self-deception. A specific sign of improvement was that near the termination of treatment he obtained a job as a salesman, a position with less immediate security but with greater potentiality for advancement.

Conventional studies of change during psychotherapy rely on a patient's conscious statements and judgments. The obvious limitation of this procedure is that significant aspects of an individual's thoughts and feelings may be immediately unverbalizable, being subject to the processes of repression and suppression. In this instance, an innovative application of the semantic differential, a method specifically designed to provide an objective measurement of the connotative aspects of meaning, was employed to supplement the more traditional objective measures of change.

The specific procedure was as follows. Prior to the waking ratings of each concept, the patient relaxed and associated about the concept for 10 minutes. The scales of the semantic differential were then read, and he responded with the values which reflected the meaning of the concept to him. He was next inducted into the hypnotic state and again asked to associate to the concept. These instructions usually evoked a spontaneous and vivid flow of thoughts and feelings which frequently gravitated to highly emotional early memories. After 10 minutes, ratings were obtained through employment of a hypnoprojective procedure designed to maintain his mood-set and to reduce his feelings of responsibility for his judgments. It was suggested that he visualize a blank movie screen with the concept to be rated at the top. He was further instructed that as the various scales were read, these would appear as if projected onto the screen and that immediately following the appearance of a scale, a small black indicator would appear at a point reflective of the generated mood state. It was

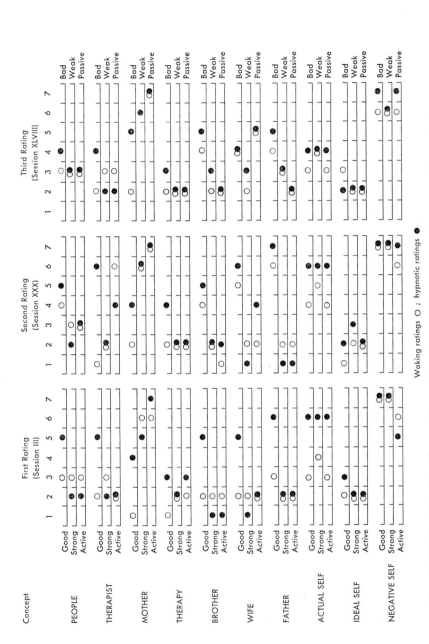

Waking ratings O ; hypnotic ratings ●

Fig. 3. Relationship of waking and hypnotic ratings of 10 concepts at three stages in psychotherapy.

emphasized that placement of the indicator would occur without volitional guidance. Questioning indicated that the patient perceived a clear visual hallucination and that the marker seemed to move without conscious direction.

Waking ratings obtained in this manner were operationally defined as a measure of "conscious" attitude and hypnotic ratings as a measure of "unconscious" meaning. Hypnotic ratings frequently had a much more negative connotation, suggesting the presence of marked ambivalence and repressed hostility. Figure 3 illustrates the relationship and movement of waking and hypnotic ratings at three stages in therapy, the three dimensions (evaluation, potency, and activity) being represented by a single pair of adjectives (actual placement is an average of ratings obtained on three sets of adjectives representing each factor). It is of interest that the change between the first and second ratings results in large part from the movement of waking (W) toward hypnotic (H) ratings (W ratings moved $D = 12.25$; H ratings moved $D = 8.31$). The change between the second and third ratings is smaller and results from the more or less equal movement of hypnotic and waking ratings (W ratings moved $D = 5.91$; H ratings moved $D = 6.78$).

Obtained data represented in Table 1 indicate a wide discrepancy between waking and hypnotic ratings at the beginning of therapy and a statistically significant reduction as treatment proceeded (the Wilcoxon Signed Ranks Test for Paired Replicates was applied to the data). The results indicate that, on the whole, hypnotic ratings are decidedly more negative in connotation than the paired waking ratings. This suggests that hypnotic ratings tap an aspect of meaning that is repressed or suppressed because of the negative valence. The therapy process seems characterized by an increasing recognition and acceptance of these negative attitudes. Demonstration that the initial increased relationship between the waking and hypnotic ratings was effected by movement of the former toward the latter suggests that previously negative attitudes are achieving an increased recognition into awareness.

TABLE 1. Distance (D² units) between hypnotic and waking ratings.

	Waking Hypnotic Distances			Differences between Sets of Distances					
	Initial Distance	Inter-mediate Distance	Final Distance	Difference	Ranks of Difference		Difference	Ranks of Difference	
Concept	$W_i - H_i$	$W_m - H_m$	$W_f - H_f$	$(W_i - H_i) - (W_m - H_m)$	+	−	$(W_i - H_i) - (W_f - H_f)$	+	−
PEOPLE	58	28	33	30	5		25	5	
MOTHER	103	72	79	31	6		24	4	
FATHER	118	43	11	75	9		107	9	
BROTHER	81	24	16	57	7		65	7	
WIFE	158	16	10	142	10		148	10	
ACTUAL SELF	103	31	30	72	8		73	8	
IDEAL SELF	13	16	15	−5		1	−2		1
NEGATIVE SELF	30	24	14	6	2		16	2	
THERAPIST	54	75	35	−21		3	19	3	
THERAPY	45	72	13	−27		4	32	6	
Σ					47	8[a]		54	1[b]

[a] Σ of divergent ranks = 8, significant at .05 level.
[b] Σ of divergent ranks = 1, significant at .01 level.

The final movement of both waking and hypnotic ratings in the direction of the initial waking ratings possibly indicates a decrease in the intensity of the negative connotative values.

Briefly, these results are tentatively interpreted to mean that areas of neurotic conflict within the personality are characterized by dissociation such that different levels of meaning, conscious and unconscious, coexist and that as conflict is resolved, there is integration of these originally discrepant levels. This interpretation is supported by the fact that, evaluated by several criteria such as psychiatric staff opinion and psychological tests, this was a successful treatment case. These data suggest that the discrepancy between conscious and unconscious attitudes obtained in this manner could provide a measure of the degree of neurotic involvement, as well as an index for improvement with psychotherapy.

A followup inquiry 10 months after formal termination revealed that the patient was reasonably satisfied with his marital and work situations and he had not felt the need for additional psychiatric assistance in the interim.

DREAMS AS AN EXPRESSION OF COVERT ATTITUDES

It has been widely maintained that dreams mirror man's innermost thoughts — feelings and attitudes that are often at variance with those expressed and even experienced in the ordinary waking state. A test of this assumption was also undertaken in this case through a comparison of the ratings of significant interpersonal concepts obtained on the semantic differential as a measure of change during psychotherapy with the attitudes expressed toward these same individuals in the patient's dreams.

The technique for obtaining the ratings of dream personages was as follows. Whenever he presented a dream, the patient was requested to rate in the waking state (prior to hypnotic examination of the symbolic meaning) the most important characters populating this dream. These waking ratings of dream personages were then compared to the most recent waking *and* hypnotic ratings of the individuals represented. The patient rated a total of 66 dream representations of one or the other of the important people in his life, and in 51 instances the ratings of the attitudes depicted in the dream were closer to the hypnotic rating of the individual represented. Instances in which the meanings of dream figures were closer to the waking ratings occurred with frequency only during the last stages of therapy when the difference between the waking and hypnotic ratings was relatively small and possibly unreliable.

These results appear to substantiate the prevalent belief that dreams express aspects of meaning outside waking awareness. The correspondence of dream with hypnotic ratings indicates that they "tap" a common abstraction of unconscious meaning. It would appear that, correctly understood, dreams do provide an important source of information concerning covert aspects of interpersonal attitudes. The fact that the patient displayed a consistency of symbolic representation and interpretation throughout therapy, despite evidence of therapeutic progress, would appear to possess some theoretical significance. That is, the resulting transparency of the symbols employed casts doubt on the psychoanalytic assumption that dream symbols are affected as a means of disguising the covert content. The stability of representation enables both patient and therapist to acquire increasing skill in the interpretation of these dreams. At the same time, despite continued exposure and practice, neither ever acquired the remarkable facility displayed by the patient in his self-induced hypnotic states.

Can it be concluded that there has been achieved a convincing demonstration of the ability of a hypnotized subject to intuit the meaning of unconsciously determined symbolism? Part of the answer depends on whether the patient relates to his own dreams or the symbols produced by other subjects. Erickson and Kubie (1940) provided the first clinical account of the ability of one hypnotized patient to intuit the symbolic modes of expression of a second patient. Farber and Fisher (1943) introduced a quasi-experimental study of the capacity of some hypnotized subjects to translate the dreams and other unconscious psychic productions of other subjects. In the concluding phase of treatment, the patient was asked to interpret three symbolic productions which possessed decided psychoanalytic (sexual and oedipal) implications. The patient in this instance was asked the meaning of two paintings, a picture of the immaculate conception featuring a snake coiled about the Madonna and a picture of St. George killing the dragon. The third stimulus was a dream presented and interpreted by another hypnotic subject.

In each instance the patient provided a highly personalized, projective interpretation. For example, in describing the first picture, he stated: "The *snake* is something which unravels from a coil — it represents my innermost thoughts and feelings and their revelation in this situation (therapy). The *Madonna* is my wife. The *picture* represents my relationship to my wife — the way in which I treated her — how she would try to get through to me but I would repulse her. The snake represents my feelings of hatred towards her and towards my parents. It shows how my wife walked into a harmful situation (marriage) unsuspecting that it was there." The dream featured a girl standing in a hallway with her boyfriend, who pressed a snake into her limp hand. Her mother eventually intervened. The girl interpreted the dream as representing the boyfriend's sexual demands upon her (refer to p. 8). The patient's interpretation was typical: "Again my wife and myself. The snake is still my 'hate' feelings and this shows how I forced them upon her and her attempt to break through my wall or barrier. She is forced to go to her mother for assistance."

If it has not been demonstrated that a hypnotized subject understands the covert content implicit in the symbolic productions of others, can it at least be concluded that hypnosis enables a subject to understand his own dreams? Several investigators have reported the ability of hypnotized subjects to understand and interpret their own dreams (Regardie, 1950; Moss, 1967b; and Sacerdote, 1967) — a moment's consideration will show the difficulty of verifying this assumption. In the only scientific investigation of this question in the past decade, Moss et al., in the chapter which follows, conclude that the interpretation of one's own dreams under the influence of hypnosis constituted a custom-tailored projective method, designed to solicit frankly projective responses from the subject. In terms of the evidence marshalled from this one intensively studied case, it seems that there is no way of establishing whether his interpretations were objective or projective — but they were seemingly *valid* in allowing him to correct his perceptions.

FOUR

The Ability
of Hypnotic Subjects
to Interpret
Symbols Generated
by Others[1]

This chapter is concerned with the hypnotic subject's ability to understand and interpret the meaning of symbolic phenomena generated by others. In the initial quasi-experimental investigation, Farber and Fisher (1943) found that approximately 20 percent of their hypnotic subjects were adept at translating a variety of symbolic content, including their own dreams and the myths, dreams, and psychotic productions of others. Perhaps the clearest statement of the affirmative position is provided by Erickson and Kubie (1940) who, in a clinical article based on the ability of one hypnotized subject to translate the cryptic automatic writing of another, conclude:

The main event of this unplanned and unexpected experience is in itself worthy of record for it is an arresting fact that one human being while in a dissociated trance-like condition can accurately decipher the automatic writing of another — writing which neither of the two subjects was able to decipher while in states of normal consciousness. The observation stresses from a new angle a fact that has often been emphasized by those who have studied unconscious processes but which remains none the less mysterious — namely, that underneath the diversified nature of the consciously organized aspects of the personality,

[1] This chapter was written and the experiments conducted by C. Scott Moss, James G. Stachowiak, and Donald E. Parente. Part of this material was originally presented in "The Ability of Hypnotic Subjects to Interpret Symbols," *Journal of Projective Techniques*, 27 (1963): 92–97. Reprinted by permission of the publisher.

the unconscious talks in a language which has laws so constant that the unconscious of one individual is better equipped to understand the unconscious of another than the conscious aspect of the personality of either (pp. 61–62).

In view of the provocative nature of this assertion, it is rather surprising that little experimentation has been undertaken in this area.

EXPERIMENTAL DATA

Study I

In 1963, Moss and Stachowiak performed the first published experimental study regarding the ability of hypnotized subjects to interpret the meaning of symbolic productions. Three test items included a fairy tale (Little Red Riding Hood), a brief Rorschach protocol, and a dream.[2] In a few instances, time permitting and where a subject showed exceptional promise of interpretative ability, two additional items were administered, a Biblical excerpt, Jonah and the whale, and a detailed example of cryptic automatic writing reported in the aforementioned article by Erickson and Kubie. These items were chosen deliberately to represent a wide range of difficulty and a variety of validating criteria. Each item was treated separately in the analysis of results, and responses were judged on the basis of (a) over-all agreement with the criterion variable and (b) the specific interpretation of seven or eight of the most prominent symbols appearing in each test item. Data were also scrutinized for communality of interpretation among subjects, regardless of "objective" correctness.

In the first phase of Study I, the three standard items were presented to 22 waking subjects for interpretation. These volun-

[2] The fairy tale was taken from Fromm's *The Forgotten Language* (1951), and his interpretation was used as the determinant of correctness. The meaning of the Rorschach protocol, chosen from a paper by Moss (1957c), had been consensually validated by three schizophrenic patients, while the dream had been produced and interpreted by a patient possessed of singular and impressive skill in interpreting his own dreams under hypnosis (Moss, 1957a).

teer college students were told that recent research had conclu-
sively demonstrated that symbolism was a highly meaningful language and that many people had an unsuspected or latent ability
to understand this form of communication. They were instructed
to avoid approaching the task in an intellectual or logical manner; instead, they were asked to relax, free-associate, and to
await spontaneous insight. While a modest range of individual
differences was obtained, there was no evidence that any subject
possessed impressive ability at symbol translation.

A sizable group of college students was next screened on the
basis of the Friedlander-Sarbin Scale of Hypnotic Suggestibility
(1938), and 15 hypnotizable subjects were selected (eight of
whom were full somnambules). Each subject was utilized as his
own control, since all test items were first presented in the waking and then in the hypnotic state for interpretation. This was a
very time-consuming procedure, of course, requiring four to five
hours per subject. Subjects were requested under both conditions
to free-associate to the item as a whole and then to selected symbols. A method designed to facilitate imaginal associations was
also used; subjects were asked to imagine a movie screen and on
it the symbol in question and they were then told that at a given
signal the symbol would be automatically replaced by a second
image, representative of the underlying, covert content (see
Chapter Two).

Results were disappointingly negative in terms of agreement
with the external validating criteria; nor did subjects demonstrate
any appreciable agreement among themselves. There were occasional insights, usually attributable to the transparency of the
symbolized content and the applicability of conventional social
stereotypes; for example, many subjects interpreted "wolf" as
meaning a predatory male, or interpreted the flight of Jonah as
an attempt to escape the wrath of God.

Study II

In the second study, nine advertisements were chosen as the
stimuli — seven were for perfume products and two for floor

wax. Two of the advertisements, one for perfume and one for floor wax, were straightforward, factual presentations. The other seven advertisements were more imaginal or ambiguous and were allegedly open to a wide variety of symbolic and nonsymbolic interpretations. For example, one advertisement showed a picture of a girl dressed as a tiger, a second showed a picture of a girl in a fencing outfit standing in a kitchen, a third showed a woman standing in front of a unicorn, and so forth (see Fig. 4).

Control and experimental groups were carefully selected. Each group consisted of 10 female undergraduate students between the ages of 19 and 23, all the subjects were volunteers, and it was established before the study that each subject was highly hypnotically suggestible. Seventeen of the subjects were full somnambules in the sense that they were capable of achieving positive hallucinations; all of the 20 subjects were able to achieve amnesia.

In the experimental group, the subjects were exposed to the nine stimuli, were asked to respond to each of the pictures with a story, and were also asked to fill out a semantic differential form on each of the pictures. They were then hypnotized, exposed to the same stimuli, and were again asked to tell a story and to fill out the semantic differential test forms. The control group was treated similarly except that they were not hypnotized until after the pre- and poststories and the tests. Specifically, both sets of subjects in the pretest waking state were instructed to "tell a story about what you see in the picture, what it represents to you." Prior to the post-test of these same advertisements in the waking or hypnotic states, subjects were instructed to close their eyes and try to imagine how their subconscious might react or feel about the ads and then to "tell a story about what you see in the picture or what it may represent to you much as you might experience it in a dream." However, in no case were the subjects actually allowed to engage in hypnotic dreaming.

Table 2 depicts the distance (D) mean score values for the experimental and control groups across each of the nine advertisements. It is of interest to note that the *differences* between the group means were greater for the experimental group in every instance. The key question is concerned with the degree of difference between the two groups: are the differences obtained from the experimental group significantly greater than those obtained from the control group? The point seems self-evident. By any statistical test, the experimental group is clearly superior in their ability to reformulate the meaning of the stories while under hypnosis in contrast to the stories told by the matched control group in the pre- and post-tests. An analysis of individual scores turned up only one extreme case, a member of the experimental group, where the difference between waking and hypnotic scores summed into the low 70's; but this would only have affected the group mean by two to three points. However, an F-test run between each set of group means yielded a statistically significant difference in only two instances. No difference was found in comparing the semantic differential ratings of the two so-called factual advertisements (6 and 8) with the symbolic or more ambiguous figures.

TABLE 2. Distance (D) score values for the experimental and control groups across advertisements with a one-way analysis of variance test (F).

| Advertisement | Group Means | | Difference | F Values |
	Experimental	Control		
1	36.2	16.8	+19.4	1.98
2	55.9	29.7	+26.2	5.26[a]
3	55.7	21.0	+34.7	4.16
4	27.6	9.2	+18.4	5.97[a]
5	23.0	13.0	+10.0	2.06
6	33.9	25.3	+ 8.6	.62
7	41.9	23.8	+18.1	1.51
8	29.1	16.6	+12.5	1.79
9	46.1	35.9	+10.2	2.16

[a] Significance at .05 level = 4.41.

In this second study we were primarily interested in the differences in semantic differential scores as an objective measure of change; however, we did take down the highlights of each subject's responses to the picture. Table 3 reflects how one typical subject responded to the advertisements in the waking and the hypnotic states. Table 4 represents a cross-section of the experimental subjects' reactions to three of the advertisements. One can safely conclude that the experimental group achieved no uniformity about the nature of their stories.[3]

TABLE 3. A subject's waking and hypnotic interpretations
of the nine advertisements.

Waking	*Hypnotic*
1. The girl's lost and afraid. She has been running. She is afraid there is going to be a storm. She looks terrible. I don't like the whole picture. She is very messed up.	1. I'd like to be that girl. She is wild and free. She keeps running and never stops — goes in all kinds of weather. She looks free and contented. She just doesn't care. She's completely satisfied.
2. The cat sees something he wants but he also sees his master. She sees some object but is now sitting tight until her master leaves the room. I like the picture — especially because of the cat.	2. I would like to be a cat — be as agile as they are. I'd claw at people I don't like and rub against people that I do like. I like cats.
3. A wealthy lady — she's standing outside. A horse is behind her. She is very lonesome. Her husband leaves her alone too much. She's thinking about her life, if she was married to someone else. I don't like the picture because she's so sad. She's also arrogant. I dislike her looks. She's too dumb to have responsibility for an animal.	3. I'd like to be that lady for about a month — to be that wealthy. However, once you are wealthy you have nothing to dream for. It would be nice to have people work for you. But I don't think she's really that happy.
4. A girl in her bedroom. She is sitting in bed thinking about last night's date. She's indifferent. The dumb picture doesn't have any influence on me. She had a good time, but she's not sure if she wants to go out with him again. It's a stupid pose with her knees up. And I don't like her hair either.	4. A girl who is not afraid to do anything; she has no limitations, no restrictions on herself. She's thinking about some of the things she's done. She has no regrets because she had fun and that is the most important thing. I like her but she wouldn't be a good friend — she's not my type.

[3] The data were subjected to a factor analysis concerning all scales across all subjects, amounting to 2,880 observations. The results were reasonably similar to the original finding on the semantic differential. Four of the scales were highly loaded on the evaluation factor: beautiful-ugly, good-bad, unfriendy-friendly, and disapproval-approval; three of the scales were loaded on the activity factor: relaxed-tense, warm-cool, and sharp-dull; and two of the bipolar terms were heavily loaded on the potency factor: strong-weak and soft-hard.

TABLE 3. *Continued*

Waking	*Hypnotic*
5. A girl taking a shower. Someone comes into her bedroom and calls her. She has her mouth open and she is telling her to wait a moment; she has to have a few more clothes on. She looks friendly. I don't like the color.	5. A lady that is married and has children. She has worked hard all day so she is taking a shower. She is a very happy and contented woman. I like her. She is a good mother. I'd like to have her as a neighbor. She would assist you if you needed help.
6. Two ladies are having a discussion about floor wax. They're not really mad. They are nice ladies and have big families. They pass along hints to each other and they don't like lipstick and nail polish. They look friendly.	6. Housewives discussing floor cleaner. They take pride in their floors. Would be nice to have them as neighbors. They appear very friendly. Nice to have coffee with. I like them.
7. It is the afternoon and she has all of her housework done. She is getting ready to go out and take fencing lessons. Her kids are in school. She looks like she thinks she is above other people. A wealthy lady. She doesn't seem to care for the more exciting ideas. They [the advertisers] should use something a little more common.	7. A wealthy woman who just came home from fencing. She is proud of herself. Her instructor told her she was very good. I would like to be her. She does well in class. She is really quite out of the ordinary. That would be nice for awhile to experience great wealth.
8. I don't like it. I don't like the symmetry. It's too ordinary, too drab, too unexciting. I'd rearrange it. It needs color or people or animals in it.	8. I don't like it. I'd rearrange it somehow. It's not exciting; it's dull and ugly.
9. A jungle woman. It has a very mysterious mood. She's out to do something wrong, to destroy. I don't like it. Perhaps she will destroy some weak and helpless little animal to show her powers. It isn't at all appropriate for perfume. I don't like her hair, the claws, her expression.	9. I might like to be that woman for an hour. I wouldn't like to destroy but I would like to hurt a few people, not animals. I would have the power and the excuse if I were a jungle woman, otherwise I wouldn't normally do anything.

TABLE 4. Illustrations of differences in content by subjects reacting to three advertisements.

Waking	*Hypnotic*
Advertisement No. 3	
Jean:	
She is very sexy because of her dress and hair, but she looks cheap. I don't	She is very beautiful but sort of cheap, sort of deceiving. She acts like the most

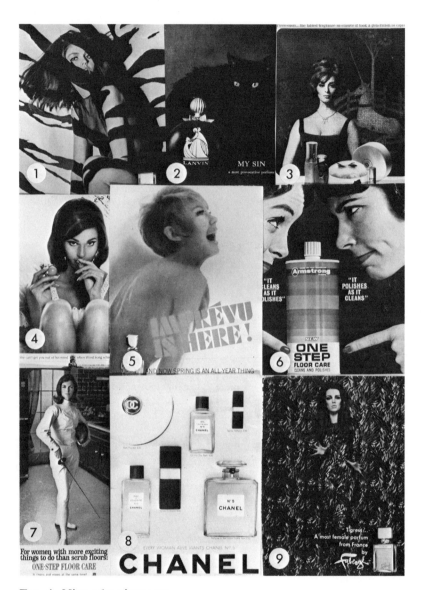

Fɪɢ. 4. Nine advertisements.

TABLE 4. *Continued*

Waking	*Hypnotic*

Advertisement No. 3

like the background, it looks out of place. It looks like a painting.

beautiful woman in the world; she has a smirk on her face and I don't like women like that.

Cathy:
This is a sophisticated woman who can catch any guy she wants. She is not trying to entice men, but she already shows some success.

The woman is alluring; she knows the ways of the world. She can see right through a male. The white steed is behind a fence, indicating his captivity. This indicates her power. The look of contentment on the horse means that this is what the male is really looking for.

Cheryle:
It doesn't look like a tree but it has daisies and a unicorn. She is a pretty rich widow, nicely talented, she wants a special kind of person — likes unicorns because they are special.

She is cold, aloof, superior, obvious. She uses people. She was born in an orphanage. She is determined to get where she is going by using people.

Advertisement No. 4

Gerry:
I like her, she's cute. She's in bed, sort of soft looking. She just got a Christmas present. But the bottle destroys the ad. It's too regal; this is not a regal situation. She is devilish in a nice sort of way. She will guile you into her bed.

She's nice because she's soft, devilish, but wicked. She likes to have fun. She just got a present. I like the ruffles on her nightgown. I'd like to be her.

Jean:
She is shy, real relaxed. She has pretty eyes. I like it except in the upper right-hand corner. Is that a broken glass? Looks like she is studying something.

She's pretty. She is trying to act shy, but she is deceiving, has an innocent look, but actually she is thinking of men. She thinks men will do things for her without having to return the favor. Maybe she tells them she is in trouble, and they give her money. I don't like deceiving women. She wants to hurt or use somebody.

Roz:
She won't forget you if you give her a gift. She is sitting in bed. I don't like the ad. Her knees — I would get sick if the ad were any lower. She's half exposed, she has fat calves, in very unflattering position. It probably appeals to men.

She's sitting in a funny position, with her legs up. Someone is looking at her. She is just leading him on, teasing him, laughing that she can get someone excited. She's half undressed. I don't like her. She's snotty.

TABLE 4. *Continued*

Waking	Hypnotic

Advertisement No. 9

Jean:

I don't like it. All blotched together. I don't like it. I don't like her eyes. Looks awful. I don't see how they could use it as an advertisement for perfume. I don't like it, period.

A tiger woman, wild, deceiving, horrible fingernails or claws. Might be ready to attack somebody, to hurt them. She likes to see pain. She's on some kind of drug — dull eyes. She's trying to be sexy but can't be. Maybe she's from India or Africa. Reminds me of those voodoo queens.

Winky:

Wild! I really like it. She's not really in the jungle — she's at a costume party. Her nails are uncovered and she's out to get a man. Really, she's not as mean as she looks. She looks so evil. I think her fingernails are a bit too long. She is studying some prey — a man.

She is in the jungle, a real animal, like a cat. She gets everything she wants. She is the queen of the jungle. I dislike her nails, they are too piercing.

Judy:

I love her nails. It is an interesting, funny, subtle background. She's like a tiger, sexy, ready to claw or to make love. She is very emotional, passionate. The nails are a little grotesque but she does look feminine.

She is cold, not a bit friendly. She only cares about herself. Her nails are vicious. I don't like her at all, even though she is wild and sexy.

DISCUSSION

The results of the present investigations did not substantiate the assertion that hypnosis can facilitate the latent capacity of subjects for understanding the symbolic language of others. None of the subjects in these studies demonstrated an ability to translate the dreams of other people. As in the study by Finzer, Kaywin, and Hilger, reported by Gill and Brenman (1959), results did suggest, however, that the hypnotized subjects "were in closer touch with their own unconscious conflicts and unsolved problems than in the normal state" (p. 350).

The chief differences in the waking and hypnotic interpretations were that the latter showed greater embellishments, the items became more personally meaningful, and the interpretations were reported with a feeling of greater subjective "certainty." The need for "cognitive congruence" was nicely illustrated in Study I where numerous subjects offered related interpretations of different test items. Several even stated the belief that because of the perceived similarity, all items must have been produced by the same person, thus exemplifying the existence of a central thema which preoccupied them to the extent that it sought expression regardless of the specific stimulus content. A striking difference evidenced in both studies was that as the investigators pressed subjects for interpretive significance in hypnosis, sudden closures were often effected, though the responses were obviously of a highly personalized nature. Many hypnotized subjects lost their usual emotional distance from their stories, for example, incorporating themselves into the stories they were telling.

It is of interest that in the interpretation of symbolic items in Study I, the subjects' interpretations were essentially nonsexual and thus dissimilar from those obtained by Farber and Fisher in the only comparable published study. This difference is possibly attributable to the relatively simple test items used in that first experiment, some undefined variation in the hypnotic relationship (the majority of subjects in that study were males), or the stronger psychoanalytic interpretation of the earlier investigators. In contrast, the subjects' interpretations of the advertisements were almost exclusively sexualized either in the waking or hypnotic states since the items themselves were highly erotically stimulating in nature.

Another interesting difference is that Farber and Fisher reported that their subjects were unable to "make any sense" out of the symbolic content presented to them in the waking state, either before or after they were hypnotized. In this study subjects always inferred some meaning. This difference is possibly attributable to the "set" established by the instructions, namely, that subjects in this study were consistently encouraged to demonstrate such an ability in both states. It should be further pointed out that Farber and Fisher's employment of suggested posthypnotic amnesia would be directly equivalent to an implanted prohibition against interpretation, and, therefore, failure to employ posthypnotic amnesia should result (and did) in spontaneous recall for the majority of subjects and a performance level at least equal to that of the hypnotic state.

In relation to the second study, many people in the field of advertising have toyed with the idea of using hypnosis to get at the covert or "unconscious" motivation of consumers. Vance Packard in his book, *The Hidden Persuaders* (1957), stated the following:

> Hypnosis is being used in attempts to probe our subconscious to find why we buy or do not buy certain products. Ruthrauff and Ryan, the New York ad agency, has been employing a prominent hypnotist and a panel of psychologists and psychiatrists in its effort to get past our mental blockages, which are so bothersome to probers when we are conscious. The agency has found that hypnosis sharpens our power to recall. We can remember things that we couldn't otherwise remember. One place they've been using it is to try to find why we use the brand of product we do (p. 34).

So far as we know, no one has yet followed up this writing and published a definitive study in this area. Whatever the rationale of the ad makers in devising these advertisements, apparently they did not succeed in communicating any specific covert idea about a particular advertisement to the public since each of the 20 subjects responded in their semantic differential ratings by making use of almost every choice of rating. But perhaps advertisers did succeed in making their advertisements ambiguous (or symbolic?), because each person tended to project onto the advertisement his own highly personalized interpretation, especially in the hypnotic situation.

If it is assumed that a hypnotic subject is anxious to please the hypnotist and will generally do whatever he is directed to the best

of his abilities, the first experimental study should have constituted a rigorous test of his capacity to engage in symbol interpretation. The high quantity of the subjects' productiveness indicates
this motive was functioning; therefore, it is of considerable
significance that they failed to confirm the experimenters' very
positive expectations. So certain were the investigators of finding
one or two subjects talented in symbol interpretation that the
procedure reported here was initially considered only as the in-
troductory step in an effort to identify the distinguishing personality characteristics of such subjects.

The authors concur with other psychologists that because of
minimal reality commitments, dreams constitute a relatively pure
form of projection. For example, Hall (1948) compared dreams
to projective test material and concluded that dreams expressed
the more socially unacceptable content; he suggested that both
dreams and projective tests should be used in personality studies.
The symbolic and therefore the essentially ambiguous nature of
dreams dictates that the act of interpretation becomes projective
in turn. That is, when subjects (or therapists) are requested to
interpret the symbolic productions of others for the ostensible
purpose of discerning the latent content, this situation is well designed to elicit projective responses by virtue of both the ambiguous nature of the stimulus and the misdirection of attention involved.

When the dream to be interpreted emanates from a subject's
own sleep consciousness, the resulting product is a nearly perfect
projective stimulus, specifically tailored, as it were, to the individual subject. (A perfect projective situation might consist of a
self-produced and interpreted dream, if it were possible to eliminate the subject's awareness of the source of the symbolic stimulus.) The introduction of hypnosis into this situation further enhances the projective qualities of the performance, since the
hypnotherapeutic relationship is ordinarily characterized by
feelings of comfort and confidence which allow the subject to
reduce his defensive operations, and the subject can be encour-

aged to direct his attention inwardly, resulting in a blurred distinction between internal and external reality and an increase in egocentricity and frank projection.

The hypnotically produced and self-interpreted dream would thus appear to provide one highly flexible approach to the "custom-built projective method" (Forer et al., 1961). Watkins (1956) and Moss (1957b) have reported on the use of the hypnoprojective fantasy in psychotherapy as a possible variation of such an approach. This is a manner of investigation and treatment that combines tactics drawn from psychoanalytic dream interpretation, hypnosis, and projective techniques of personality appraisal. The hypnotized subject is stimulated to involve himself in an ongoing, self-directed, dreamlike fantasy — his participation is subjectively most real at the moment — and the therapist encourages him to continually develop the fantasy while avoiding direction and structure.

In conclusion it is recognized that failure to verify the original intent of these investigations may reflect inadequacies of the hypnotic technique employed, for instance, insufficient time allotted for subjects to develop the required performance. Another possible limitation relates to subject selection: the occasional dramatic cases reported in the literature may be based on the fortuitous occurrence of an exceptionally gifted subject whose impressive behavior defies replication in the experimental situation. Early in his career, Freud believed that the capacity for symbol interpretation was diagnostic of schizophrenia, but later concluded that ". . . it is simply a question of a personal gift without perceptible pathological significance" (1960, p. 351).

The possibility exists that some unsophisticated persons have a capacity for symbol translation, and this remains a contaminating variable in any experiment of this nature. Nevertheless, the firmest conclusion derivable from these studies is that no evidence was obtained that hypnosis endows the ordinary subject with a propensity for symbol interpretation in any objective sense. In the absence of objective criteria it is a moot point to ask

what any unconsciously produced symbol *really* means. However, it can be stated with certainty that the interpretation of
symbolic content, especially one's own dreams, particularly
under hypnosis, is a projective method of considerable value in
soliciting covert personality dynamics.

FIVE

Alteration of
Social Attitudes
toward Negroes[1]

Frequent studies over the past half-century have failed to demonstrate consistent differences in personality between individuals who are and those who are not hypnotically susceptible. A possibility exists that the variability among individuals is due to differences in their attitudes, expectancies, and motivations with respect to the hypnotic induction situation, although again, no significant differences at all were found in recent tests of the expectancies, transference, and identification in suggestible subjects using the semantic differential (Tostado, 1970). This chapter takes a somewhat different tack and attempts to measure the effectiveness of influencing subject attitudes toward Negroes through the medium of a hypnotically administered communication. Precision was added by conceptualizing the interaction between two variables, the concept to be influenced (NEGRO) and the source of the influence (EXPERIMENTER), within the theoretical model provided by Osgood's principle of congruity. The basic value of the experiment is a paradigm for objectifying the special influence quality of the hypnotic relationship.

Hypersuggestibility is generally identified as a major characteristic of hypnosis, and one might expect that there would be considerable research directed toward measurement of the

[1] This chapter was written by James G. Stachowiak and C. Scott Moss. It is reprinted by permission from the *Journal of Personality and Social Psychology*, 2, no. 1 (July, 1965): 77–83.

effectiveness of manipulating attitudes and behavior through the medium of hypnosis. This is not the case, however, at least not in any controlled, quantifiable sense. Orne (1962) stated that it has long been held "that hypnosis increases the control of the hypnotist over the subject; however, to our knowledge this assumption has never been put to experimental test" (p. 142). By this he meant that the role contexts in which hypnosis occurs generally possess a high degree of social control, and before it is possible to arrive at an evaluation of any increment in the degree of social control by hypnosis, it is essential to isolate this variable. Orne then went on to formulate a basic consideration: "Does hypnosis increase the amount of social control over the subject *above that which existed before the induction of hypnosis?*" (p. 143).

In this chapter, an attempt was made to objectively and quantitatively determine the effectiveness of hypnosis in altering an established social attitude. The experiment was cast in the theoretical framework of the "principle of congruity" as formulated by Osgood and Tannenbaum (1955). This principle takes into account the interactions between a *source* of influence, the *concept* to be influenced, and the *nature of the assertion* or communication made about the concept by the source. The experiment was specifically directed toward providing an answer to the following question: What is the influence of hypnosis in a situation where a subject is faced with a situation of "incongruity," such that a favorable source (in this case the experimenter-hypnotist) delivers a positive communication about a less favorable concept (NEGRO)?

METHOD

Forty male undergraduate students volunteered for a study represented only as involving hypnosis and were randomly assigned to an experimental and a control group. None of the subjects had previously experienced hypnosis.

Each subject in the experimental group was seen twice individually with a 15–18 day interval elapsing between appointments. At the beginning of the first session he rated six concepts on a form of the semantic differential: EXPERIMENTER, NEGRO, COMMUNIST, JAPANESE, JEW, and REPUBLICAN. Subjects were then given the standard hypnotic induction presented in the Stanford Hypnotic Susceptibility Scale, Form A (Weitzenhoffer and Hilgard, 1959). Just prior to arousal they were read an 11-minute statement designed to positively influence their attitudes toward Negroes. After termination of hypnosis, subjects were again asked to complete the same rating forms. At the second appointment, subjects were requested to fill out the materials once more. A code and drop-box arrangement allowed subjects to retain anonymity in all of their ratings. They were repeatedly cautioned not to discuss their experiences until a week following the second appointment.

Subjects in the control group followed the same procedure with the exception that they were not hypnotized until the conclusion of the second session, after they had completed their third set of ratings. In an effort to provide the control subjects with a time period comparable to that spent by the experimental subjects in being hypnotized, the experimenter engaged each subject in a friendly discussion of course work, vocational plans, hobbies, and so forth.

The 11-minute influence presentation which was administered to both groups was obtained largely from *The Nature of Prejudice* (Allport, 1954), and was comprised of four sections: (1) a general statement of the relationship between treatment of the Negro in the United States and our threatened position of international leadership; (2) an explanation of stereotyped beliefs and attitudes; (3) a description of how unconscious psychological mechanisms relate to prejudiced beliefs; (4) suggestion of a solution through migration and intermarriage.

Two hypotheses, derived from the congruity principle, concern the prediction of the direction and magnitude of attitude change toward the source and concept *within* the experimental and the control groups.

Hypothesis I — Direction of the attitude change. Attitude change toward a source and a concept related by an assertion will be in the direction of greater congruity.

According to one of the corollaries derived from Osgood's congruity principle, whenever two differently polarized objects of judgment are related by an associative assertion, the less polarized object of judgment becomes more polarized, and the more polarized object of judgment becomes less so (Osgood and Tannenbaum, 1955). It would thus be predicted that the NEGRO (slightly positive concept) will become more positive, and the EXPERIMENTER (quite positive source) will become less positive, if the experimenter makes a positive assertion about the Negro. It should be noted that this prediction is expected to hold for the control group but not for the experimental group, since the anticipated effect of hypnotizing the subjects would be to enhance the esteem of the experimenter, thus increasing the polarization of an already favorable source.

Hypothesis II — Magnitude of the attitude change. (a) The amount of positive attitude change toward the concept will be proportional to the degree of favorableness of the original attitude toward the source. (b) The amount of negative attitude change toward the source will be proportional to the degree of favorableness of the original attitude toward the concept.

Two additional hypotheses relate to the effects of hypnosis on the attitude changes of the subjects.

Hypothesis III. The amount and persistence of positive attitude change will be significantly greater for subjects who are exposed to a persuasive communication while they are in hypnosis.

Hypothesis IV. The amount and persistence of positive attitude change induced will be proportional to a subject's susceptibility to hypnosis.

On the basis of an assumed relationship between waking and hypnotic suggestibility, it was predicted that even among the control subjects there would be a greater positive impact of the assertion on the concept, both immediate and long term, and a lessened amount of attitude change in a negative direction toward the experimenter, for those subjects who evidenced greater hypnotic susceptibility.

RESULTS

The basic semantic differential data consisted of two sets of "difference scores" for each subject: one set was obtained by subtracting each subject's first rating of each concept from his second rating, thereby yielding an index of "immediate" attitude change. The second was obtained by subtracting the first ratings from the third ratings, providing a measure of the "persistence" of the induced attitude change.

To test whether the change scores on the four control concepts differed significantly from one another, the Friedman two-way analysis of variance for related samples was applied. Analyses were not significant and these scores were then pooled within each group in order to next determine whether the subjects' change scores for EXPERIMENTER and NEGRO were significantly different from the means of their change scores for the control concepts. The Wilcoxon Signed Ranks Test for Paired Replicates was employed and results are presented in Table 5.

For the experimental group the mean change score for the concept NEGRO was significantly more positive than the mean change score for the control concepts, for both sets of scores. For the control group, the change scores for NEGRO did not differ significantly, but change scores for EXPERIMENTER were significantly more negative than the means of the change scores for the control concepts on both sets of ratings.

From Hypothesis I it was predicted that, for the control group, immediate attitude change would be in a positive direction for NEGRO and in a negative direction for EXPERIMENTER. For the experimental group, it was predicted that change toward both

TABLE 5. Differences between change scores for the experimental and control concepts.

Index		Change Score	Wilcoxon Z
Experimental Group			
NEGRO vs. mean of control concepts	Ratings I–II		2.40[a]
	Ratings I–III		2.33[a]
EXPERIMENTER vs. mean of control concepts	Ratings I–II		1.29
	Ratings I–III		.95
Control Group			
NEGRO vs. mean of control concepts	Ratings I–II		.04
	Ratings I–III		.52
EXPERIMENTER vs. mean of control concepts	Ratings I–II		3.77[b]
	Ratings I–III		3.33[c]

Note: All probabilities are one-tailed and significant differences are in the direction: NEGRO > mean of control concepts for the experimental group; EXPERIMENTER < mean of control concepts for the control group.
[a] $p < .01$.
[b] $p < .0001$.
[c] $p < .001$.

NEGRO and EXPERIMENTER would be in a positive direction. The predicted direction of change was confirmed in all four cases. It can be seen in Fig. 5 that the original location of EXPERIMENTER on the seven-step semantic differential grid was approximately

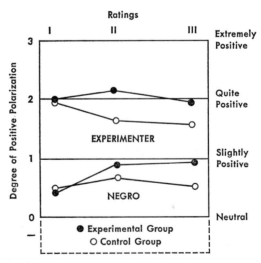

FIG. 5. Means of the three ratings of EXPERIMENTER and NEGRO on the semantic differential for the experimental and control groups.

the same for both groups, and the resulting attitude change was in opposite directions for the experimental and control groups. The original location of NEGRO was slightly more favorable for the control group than for the experimental group; however, the greater obtained change in the experimental group resulted in NEGRO becoming more favorable for this group.

The observation of greater congruity between attitudes held toward EXPERIMENTER and toward NEGRO can be demonstrated even more strikingly by comparing the amount of distance between each subject's ratings of these concepts on the semantic differential for Ratings I, II, and III. It would be expected that the amount of distance would tend to be smaller on Ratings II and III (after exposure to the communication) than the amount of distance present before exposure to the communication. The results are presented in Table 6.

TABLE 6. Analysis of the change in amount of distance between ratings of EXPERIMENTER and NEGRO on the semantic differential.

Index	Wilcoxon Z
Experimental Group	
Ratings I–II	1.45
Ratings I–III	2.31[a]
Control Group	
Ratings I–II	3.70[b]
Ratings I–III	2.56[c]

[a] $p < .05$.
[b] $p < .0001$.
[c] $p < .01$.

The highly significant results for the control group lend considerable support for Hypothesis I. The analysis for Ratings I-II within the experimental group also approach significance at the .07 level.

Two specific predictions were made concerning the amounts of change to be expected toward NEGRO and toward EXPERIMENTER. First, it was hypothesized that the amount of positive change toward NEGRO should be proportional to the degree of favorableness of the original attitude toward EXPERIMENTER. This prediction was tested by applying the Spearman rank-correlation coefficient. The results were in the predicted direction for both the experimental and the control groups, but neither of the coefficients reaches significance.

With respect to predicted amounts of change toward EXPERIMENTER, the resulting coefficients were again in a positive direction but quite negligible in magnitude. Thus, there appeared to be no significant relationship between the subject's original attitudes toward NEGRO and the amount of obtained change toward EXPERIMENTER.

An analysis of the scores obtained on the Stanford Hypnotic Susceptibility Scale for the subjects within both the experimental and control groups revealed no significant difference in the hypnotic susceptibility of the two groups. Both groups averaged above the Stanford norms, the mean for the experimental group being 7.10 and for the control group, 7.05. In each group 50 percent of the subjects scored between 8 and 12 on the Stanford Scale, which is the interval assigned to highly susceptible individuals.

It was expected that the experimental and control groups would differ significantly with respect to the amount and persistence of the obtained positive attitude changes toward EXPERIMENTER and toward NEGRO. The results are presented in Table 7.

It can be seen that the amounts of immediate positive attitude change toward EXPERIMENTER and NEGRO are significantly greater for the experimental than for the control group. With respect to EXPERIMENTER, this means that while the attitudes of the control group become *less* favorable, the attitudes of the experimental group become slightly *more* favorable. With respect to NEGRO, both groups change in a positive direction, but the amount was significantly greater for the experimental group.

Analyses with respect to persistence of attitude change again revealed that the two groups differed significantly. While attitude change toward NEGRO remained substantially stable for the experimental group, it diminished for the control group, with the attitudes returning to their original location on the semantic differential grid. It should be noted that the experimental subjects' attitudes toward EXPERIMENTER became slightly less favorable than they were originally. The finding of a significant difference between the experimental and control groups, however, results from the fact that the latter group tended to become even less favorable than they were directly after being exposed to the persuasive communication.

TABLE 7. Comparison of the amount and persistence of positive attitude change toward EXPERIMENTER and NEGRO for the experimental and control groups.

Concept	Difference between Groups (Mann-Whitney Z)
Ratings I–II	
EXPERIMENTER	2.85[a]
NEGRO	1.76[b]
Ratings I–III	
EXPERIMENTER	1.89[b]
NEGRO	1.69[b]

Note: In all cases, the direction of difference is experimental > control.
[a] $p < .005$.
[b] $p < .05$.

It was predicted that both the amount and persistence of positive attitude change would be proportional to the degree of hypnotic susceptibility. The Spearman coefficient (rho) was again utilized in order to obtain a measure of the association between the various sets of variables. In terms of immediate alterations in attitude there was only one significant change: for the control group there was a negative correlation with respect to change toward EXPERIMENTER and hypnotic susceptibility beyond the .01 level. Such a finding suggests that while the amount of change induced may be proportional to a subject's hypnotic susceptibility, the direction of change is not readily predictable from the nature of the influence attempt.

For the experimental group the persistence of change toward

NEGRO correlated with hypnotic susceptibility beyond the .05 level, and the correlation between persistence of change toward EXPERIMENTER and hypnotic susceptibility approaches significance ($p = .06$). The coefficients for the control group did not reach significance in this instance.

All concepts with the exception of EXPERIMENTER were also rated on a modified form of the Bogardus Social Distance Scale. It had orginally been planned to submit change scores on these to analyses similar to those undertaken for the change scores on the semantic differential. It was found, however, that the ordering of the concepts along the scale by the subjects was highly similar for both groups, with little change from one rating to another. Although the original rankings of the concepts remained quite stable and resistant to change, it should be noted that the change in ratings of NEGRO for the experimental subjects was greater than the change in ratings on any of the other concepts for either group.

DISCUSSION

A major corollary derived from Osgood's theory is that if two positive but unequally polarized concepts are associated by a positive assertion, the less polarized should become more polarized and the more polarized concept less so. In the present investigation the effect of introducing the variable of hypnosis into this situation altered the ordinarily obtained results in both the experimental and control groups; that is, in the former both the concepts NEGRO and EXPERIMENTER changed in a positive direction, while in the latter there was a marked decrease in the positive connotation of EXPERIMENTER. All changes were in the predicted direction, however, in accordance with the expected effects of hypnosis upon the esteem of the experimenter.

Hypothetically, the effect of hypnotizing the subjects was to increase the degree of positive polarization for EXPERIMENTER, and his positive communication about NEGRO created a greater pressure toward congruity than was present in the control group, since the distance between attitude ratings toward EXPERIMENTER and NEGRO was presumably greater at this point. The positive attitude toward NEGRO persisted over the two-week interval, despite a decline in favorableness toward EXPERIMENTER. Further research would be necessary in order to clarify this effect.

Some insufficiencies are evident with regard to predictions of the magnitude of the obtained attitude changes. While changes in direction were all as predicted, the magnitude of changes in both groups was small (on the average much less than one scale unit), and consequently it could not be demonstrated that the amount of change for either concept was proportional to the original attitude toward the other concept. According to Osgood's theory, one would predict that the less polarized object, NEGRO, should change more than the more polarized, EXPERIMENTER. For the control group, however, the mean attitude change in a negative direction toward EXPERIMENTER was almost twice as large as the change in a positive direction toward NEGRO.

In reviewing the data, Osgood raised the question of whether the obtained original ratings of NEGRO were an adequate representation of the subjects' "true" feelings. That is, if the "true" original locus of NEGRO on the semantic differential grid was − 2, the obtained change would be in close agreement with the change predicted by the congruity principle. This raises the possibility of using congruity shifts as estimates of subjects' "true" attitudes toward socially legitimized concepts. However, there was no way to check further on the validity of the subjects' attitudes.

It may be that the degree of polarization cannot be directly equated with resistance to change as postulated by Osgood: for example, an individual may hold an "intensely neutral" attitude. Another explanation is that waking subjects are less receptive to directive attempts to manipulate their attitudes, and displayed their resentment by discrediting the source but not the object of the assertion. A third plausible explanation resides in the fact that subjects volunteered with an expectation of being hypnotized. The negative reaction of the control group toward the experimenter could be attributable to an experience of disappointment over not being hypnotized at once. It is noteworthy that those who developed the strongest negative reaction were subsequently demonstrated to possess the highest tested hypnotic susceptibility. Needed to clarify this issue is a third group in which this factor of expectation is controlled by avoidance of any mention of hypnosis, or a group of subjects who are hypnotized but not given the influencing message. It would also have illumined the situation if the control group could have ultimately had exposure to the assertion during their experience in hypnosis.

One final, important factor, directly relevant to the present study, is that the congruity principle does not provide adequately for differences in the complexity and the degree of intensity of the assertion made by the source. An assertion is identified merely as being "associative" or dissociative." A deliberate attempt was made in the present experiment, for example, to develop a strong, favorable, rational communication about the Negro. However, the experimenter's stated position on intermarriage may have served to place the focus of the communication on the experimenter in a negative fashion for some of the subjects. They may have experienced the experimenter as putting them in a "double-bind," with the result being that they responded in a contradictory or ambivalent fashion. It should be noted that this is not unlike the situation frequently encountered in psychotherapy, where the therapist's assertions (interpretations) are often complex and involved and may be met with considerable ambivalence on the part of the patient. In any case, further research on the nature and intensity of the assertion is definitely indicated.

The predictions concerning the increased effectiveness of presenting the persuasive communication to subjects in hypnosis were generally confirmed, with respect to both immediate and persisting changes in attitude. However, the expected correlation between the degree of measured susceptibility to hypnosis and the amount and persistence of attitude change was not substantiated. There is apparently no simple and direct relationship between these two behaviors. These results would appear to be consistent with the conclusions of experienced hypnotherapists, such as Gill and Brenman (1959), who state "there is no correlation between the depth of hypnosis obtainable in a patient and the therapeutic results" (p. 333). The mere fact of being subjected to a formal hypnotic procedure seems sufficient to increase the persuasibility of some subjects, independent of the degree of hypnotic susceptibility as measured on an instrument such as the Weitzenhoffer-Hilgard scale. Hilgard (personal communication) has suggested the possibility that "the general attitude of relaxation and detachment, giving one's attention to the hypnotist, is what matters, and an interesting control would be to use people simulating hypnosis in the same situation." It could thus be determined whether persons simulating hypnosis would also be susceptible to the social influence procedure, even though they themselves were not (strictly speaking) hypnotized.

The inability to obtain significant changes in ratings on the Bogardus scale suggests that this circumscribed influence attempt might be expected to have little or no effect on the subject's actual behavior with respect to minority groups such as Negroes. The semantic differential measurement technique is apparently more sensitive to small or restricted changes than the gross units of the Bogardus scale. At the same time, however, the Bogardus scale may be considered to be closer to the "action level"; that is, it is more directly related to how a person might actually behave in social situations. It is relatively easy for a person to report a change in his attitudes without necessarily changing his behavior. Then, too, it is important to emphasize that in the present study it was in no way suggested that the subjects were to "change" their behavior. Being "good hypnotic subjects" they may be considered to have performed quite literally in accordance with the hypnotist's suggestions.

Although this is a sensitive area and ethical considerations are involved, it would be of interest to attempt to increase the magnitude of the presently obtained attitude changes through repeated inductions with the same subjects. While it is possible that this might result in a greater degree of change in attitude and behavior itself, it could just as easily affect a subject's receptivity to the experience of being hypnotized, i.e., the resistance to hypnosis mounting as the attitude toward the experimenter-hypnotist goes down. The hypnotic interpersonal relationship is highly involved, and the question of the hypnotist's assertions and their reception is a matter of extreme importance for future research.

The effort to educate and indoctrinate, to alter and influence behavior, is a paramount feature of human social intercourse. Most experiments in this area have involved simple measurement of the *magnitude* of change as a function of *gross* content. Osgood's principle of congruity provided a theoretical framework for isolating and measuring with considerable exactness the interaction between the *source* of an assertion about specific *concepts*. While it is difficult to generalize from the relatively simple experiment reported here to specific problems in everyday life, there is obvious possible extension to such situations as psychotherapy.

It seems demonstrated that, as frequently maintained, hypnosis precipitates a special rapport or transference reaction, although the exact nature of the relationship remains to be established. To many modern-day psychotherapists the employment of suggestion, particularly in association with hypnosis, is anathema. Yet, psychotherapy is in essence only a professionalized effort to persuade people to adopt new ideas and different ways of behaving. Whether or not the clinician approves, suggestion, direct and covert, is an integral and important aspect of the therapeutic relationship (Frank, 1961). Thus, Alexander and French (1946) have stated that, "Methodical psychotherapy is, to a large degree, nothing more than the systematic conscious application of those methods by which we influence our fellow man" (p. viii). No substantial progress can be made in evaluating the efficacy of the many competing systems of psychotherapy until the pervasive common element of suggestion is isolated and controlled. This chapter presents a basic method of broad applicability for objectifying this important aspect of the psychotherapeutic transaction.

SIX

Homogeneity
of Szondi Test
Classifications[1]

INTRODUCTION

It may be recalled that in the early 1930's a Hungarian psychiatrist, Lipot Szondi, developed a genetic theory of personality predicated on the existence of drives which arise from the vectorial opposition of pairs of needs whose strength is genetically determined. He postulated the existence of four drive vectors (sexual, paroxysmal, schizophrenia, and contact), each of which embraces two clinically definable reaction types. In 1937, Szondi advanced a personality test derived from his theory allowing classification of subjects under one or another of these eight drive-needs. Borstelmann and Klopfer (1953) describe the Szondi Test as follows:

The Szondi Test materials consist of 48 facial photographs of European psychiatric patients, with six representatives of each of eight diagnostic categories: passive male homosexuals, male sadistic murderers, epileptics in the intraparoxysmal phase, hysterics, catatonic schizophrenics, manic depressives in the depressive and in the manic phases. The test pictures are arranged into six sets, each containing one picture from each of the eight diagnostic groups (position of a given category within the set is randomized). The sets are administered successively to the subject with instructions to select the two "most liked" and the two "most disliked" pictures from each set. The

---

[1] This chapter was written by Stephen S. Baratz and C. Scott Moss.

This study is the only one that does not use hypnosis per se and is included here because of the relationship between projective techniques and dreams, and because it testifies to the sensitive screening of the semantic differential measurements.

90

subject thus has six opportunities to like, dislike, or ignore each class of pictures. The resulting pattern of 24 choices (12 likes and 12 dislikes) is represented by an eight-dimension profile.

Szondi's genetic theory met with little acceptance in the United States, but considerable speculation and research was stimulated in relation to the question of what a subject's choices reflect about the process mediating between the stimulus pictures and his personality. Most of the research on the Szondi Test was concerned with the stimulus properties of the photographs. A major proportion of studies dealt either with the ability of subjects to match individual pictures in accordance with Szondi's diagnostic groupings or to determine the homogeneity of stimulus value of pictures within particular categories. Since Deri's (1949) introduction of the test into the United States, four major critical reviews of the experimental literature have appeared: Guertin and McMahan (1951), Deri (1952), Borstelmann and Klopfer (1953), and Aumack (1957).

A rapidly diminishing interest in the clinical application of the Szondi Test or even as a focus for research is mirrored in the fact that while the *Fourth Mental Measurements Yearbook* (1953) listed 64 references to the test and the fifth edition (1959) listed 74, the most recent (1965) volume contained only 21 additional references through 1962. Similarly, the *Psychological Abstracts* lists only six studies (1962–63) and none at all have appeared for the past five years. This chapter, concerned with the issue of whether or not the test item photographs are unique in the *constituted categories* so as to be defferentiable from one another, might well represent a final footnote to the history of one more interesting psychological test.

EXPERIMENTAL DESIGN

Questions to Be Evaluated

1) Do Szondi's eight diagnostic categories differ from one another with respect to average "stimulus value"?

2) In particular, do the two diagnostic categories which define the ends of any of Szondi's four vectors differ in "stimulus value"?

Measuring Device

The principal measuring instrument employed in evaluation of the Szondi Test was a form of the semantic differential. The first use of the semantic differential to isolate and identify the latent stimulus properties of various projective test instruments was Reeves' (1954) evaluation of the TAT. Since that time there have been over two dozen studies of different projective tests using the semantic differential. The nine semantic scales employed in the present study were selected as representative of three factors identified in Osgood's original factor analytic study, the evaluation, potency, and activity dimensions.

Procedure

Thirty college student subjects met in small groups in which the Szondi Test was administered via slides projected on a screen in the order prescribed by Szondi. Each picture was then judged by each subject independently on a separate page of a 48-page semantic differential booklet. The results of this single administration were coded onto IBM cards for analysis. The ratings of individual pictures constituting a Szondi category were pooled on the assumption that the dynamics underlying each picture within a Szondi category were similar.

RESULTS

The data were first cast into an analysis of variance design allowing analysis of the interaction of semantic differential factors and Szondi categories. When pooled across subjects and semantic differential categories, it was found that the Szondi categories differ significantly ($p < .001$). Shaffe's (1953) test, using mean differences as the comparison statistic, indicates that out of 28 possible Szondi category comparisons, the differences in 11 prove to be significant at the .01 level, while four additional differences are significant at the .05 level. Thus some of Szondi's eight diagnostic categories seem to differ significantly from each other in stimulus value.

TABLE 8. Summary of category comparisons.

	h	s	e	hy	k	p	d	m
h	—							
s	.05	—						
e	ns	ns	—					
hy	ns	.05	ns	—				
k	ns	.01	.05	ns	—			
p	.01	ns	.01	.01	.01	—		
d	ns	.01	.05	ns	ns	.01	—	
m	.01	ns	ns	.01	.01	ns	.01	—

In relation to question two, which concerns Szondi's assumption that the two diagnostic categories defining the ends of any of the four vectors will have contrasting stimulus values, only the paroxysmal vector, composed of the hysteric and epileptic categories, failed to provide a significant difference. That is, significant differences occur in the sexual vector ($p < .01$ between the paranoid and catatonic categories) and the contact vector ($p < .01$ between the depressive and manic categories).

When the Szondi category means were considered in light of the semantic factor scores, a significant factor-by-category interaction effect was noted ($p < .001$). In order to determine which specific dimensions contributed most to these category differences, Shaffe's test was next applied to the mean differences with the following results.

Sexual vector. The homosexual pictures differ from the sadist pictures significantly by being perceived as *less potent.*

Paroxysmal vector. No significant differences.

Schizophrenic vector. Out of eight significant differences in the evaluation factor, seven of these occur in comparisons with this vector, and it is the paranoid category which accounts for six of the positive ratings ("most liked").

TABLE 9. Summary of factor-by-category comparisons.[a]

	h	s	e	hy	k	p	d	m
h	—							
s	Po	—						
e	Po	ns	—					
hy	ns	ns	ns	—				
k	ns	Po	ns	ns	—			
p	Ev	Ev	Ev	Ev	Ev	—		
d	ns	Po	ns	ns	ns	Ev Ac	—	
m	Po	ns	ns	ns	Ev	ns	Ev	—

[a] All factor-by-category differences are significant at the .05 level.
Ev = evaluation; Po = potency; Ac = activity.

Contact vector. The manic and depressive categories are complete opposites. The manic category differs from the homosexual on the potency factor, while its vectorial opposite, the depressive, differs from the vectorial opposite, the sadist, on the same semantic factor. Furthermore, in terms of semantic factors, while there is no significant difference on the paroxysmal vector, the within-vector differences for the contact vector are always on the same factors.

Not only do the manic and depressive categories differ from each other, but they align themselves selectively with the opposite categories of every other vector. The depressive member of the contact vector differs from the paranoid member of the schizophrenic vector on the evaluation and activity dimensions, while the manic member of the contact vector differs from the catatonic member on the evaluation dimension only. Examination of Table 8 reveals a trend in the direction of selective alignment throughout all of the vectorial combinations. As can be seen from Table 9, two other category differences were observed (epileptic: homosexual; paranoid: sadist) which did not demonstrate significant category differences but do differ significantly when their factor differences are considered. Figure 6 presents the mean semantic factor scores on each vector.

The analysis to this point has been restricted to the profiles, and it is possible to place each category on a *continuum of in-*

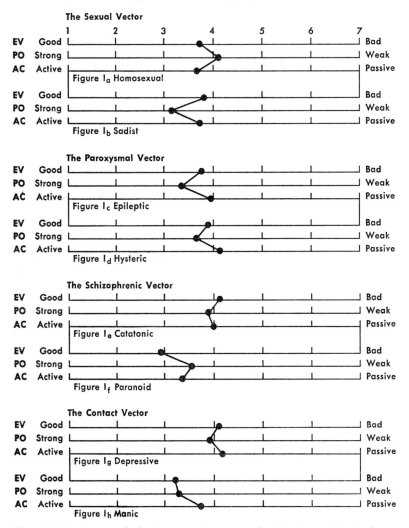

FIG. 6. Mean semantic factor scores by categories. Each score in the figure is the mean of the three component semantic differential scales for that factor.

tensities regardless of differences in the three semantic factors. Figure 7 depicts each category in its relative position to other categories. Visual inspection reveals two distinct groupings. The first group includes the paranoid, manic, sadist, and epileptic categories; the second, the hysteric, homosexual, catatonic, and depressive categories. As is immediately apparent, each group contains one component category of each of the four Szondi vectorial pairs. Further inspection of the same figure reveals that the depressive category shows significant differences only from those categories in Group One, while the manic category shows significant differences only from those categories in Group Two. Both the depressive and the manic categories belong to the contact vector.

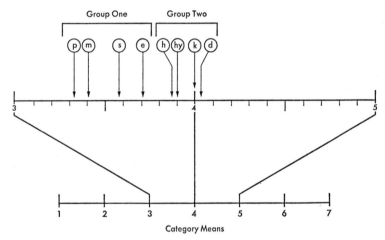

FIG. 7. Graphic distribution of category means.

DISCUSSION

Implications for Szondi Test Interpretations

The single most important finding was that 15 of a possible 28 comparisons of differences between categories proved to be significant, a finding which lends support to Szondi's assertion that no two categories are alike. His contention that the component members of each of the four vectorial pairs differ from each other was also supported in three of the four comparisons.

Furthermore, it was within the sexual vector that all of the significant potency differences occurred. Consistent with Szondi's speculations, the sadist category was perceived as the most potent while the homosexual category was seen as least potent. Szondi considered that the schizophrenic vector reflected ego functioning whereby needs are bound and assimilated into meaningful action. While findings provide no direct confirmation of this interpretive assumption, it is within this vector that seven of the eight significant differences on the evaluation factor were obtained. It would appear that this is the vector which normal subjects most clearly differentiate on an evaluative basis, and of all the Szondi categories, they tend to identify with the paranoid (as "best liked") and to dissociate themselves from the catatonic (as "least liked").

As was noted, the components of the contact vectors selectively align themselves with the opposing categories in each of the other vectors, forming two distinct groups. It would appear that all four categories in Group One share a marked externalizing mode of expression of need; on the other hand, Group Two seems to share in a more subtle, inward, passive form of reactivity. It is concluded that the contact vector seems to differentiate between an externalizing and an internalizing mode of adjustment, reflecting a significant difference in the orientation of the individual to himself and to others. That is, not only are each of the vectors composed of opposing needs, but the principle of opposition seems similar for the four vectors. This principle may be very tentatively described in terms of an *internalization-externalization* dichotomy.

The paroxysmal vector (epileptic and hysteric) was the only one in which the stimulus intensities of both categories were insufficiently different to bear out Szondi's contention of polarity of needs within this vector. The reason for this failure of differentiation appears to lie within the epileptic category. While the epileptic category resides well within Group One, it is unique because it is the only category of the eight which shares differences with some of the "Internalizers" and some of the "Externalizers." This category stands at the mid-point on the intensity scale. At the same time, the vector itself is most elusive of empirical description, as Borstelmann and Klopfer also found, and should be investigated further.

Implications for Future Research

These findings seem inconsistent with the essentially negative results of many previous studies. However, most of the negative results have derived from investigations which treated the stimulus pictures in terms of communalities extracted from the pictures themselves (e.g., traits, free associations, and so forth). Results of the present study suggest that there is a shared stimulus value, observable when pictures are pooled into their categories but not when the individual pictures are treated separately.

It should be noted that this study is a partial replication of that of Rabin (1950), who found that subjects could match diagnostic labels with the pictures with better than chance occurrence. The present investigation suggests that subjects can perform the task of sorting the pictures into the designated categories without recourse to the diagnostic labels. One of the problems not confronted in this experiment was whether the variance between categories was greater than that within categories; that is, could the results be attributable to only one or two pictures within each category?

Another consideration is that the Szondi Test instructions may have had a contaminating effect on the semantic differential ratings. The greatest factor loading on the semantic differential occurs on the evaluation factor, and when used above, this factor in effect constitutes an attitude scale. When, as in this study, subjects are instructed first to designate most "liked" and "disliked" choices and then to rate them on the semantic differential, the possibility exists that the significance of the potency and activity factors may be diminished. Subjects might tend to regard the rating task as a simple evaluative exercise. For this reason the study should be repeated and the rating of the pictures should be obtained prior to eliciting statements of preference for the photographs.

While this study assiduously avoided treating the pictures apart from their categories, it remains to discuss a method whereby the relationship of the individual Szondi pictures to their categories might be determined. This objective could be achieved by identification through a large-scale sampling of dichotomous semantic terms, those adjectives which are specifically relevant to the Szondi pictures. Szondi has given an assist in this task by dividing the eight categories into the four vectors. In addition, the present results suggest that there is a common base around which the vectors themselves seem to relate, i.e., "Internalizers-Externalizers." Working with this dichotomy it should be possible to construct rating scales from a factor analytic study of our sample of dichotomous terms. These rating scales might then be utilized to articulate the relationship of the individual picture to the category. The individual pictures within a category should have somewhat similar scores within the category and differ from other pictures not in the category.

In conclusion, psychologists in this past decade have somewhat lost interest in projective techniques, and this chapter is a historical postscript to a test which has met with a sudden demise in clinical interest. The results are not so astonishing if the reasonable assumption is made that Lipot Szondi carefully selected the photographs constituting his test on the basis of some predetermined physiognomic criteria as well as an explicit personality theory. A series of carefully designed studies could eventually succeed in teasing out the physical characteristics which Szondi assumedly used to organize his test, the proven existence of which would, of course, have no reference whatsoever to the validity of his theoretical postulates.

SEVEN

Experimental Aspects of Dream Symbolism

The central importance of meaning in personality study and psychotherapy cannot be overemphasized. Many authors have tried to define a personality trait and they end up with the statement that it is essentially a central event which renders equivalent a class of situations and a class of related behaviors, so that it renders all of these situations functionally equivalent in terms of mediating a variety of behaviors. For example, a trait of inferiority is solicited in any situation which involves competition with other people; such circumstances will have a certain significance to a person which is somewhat different from the significance of the situation to other individuals not possessed of the trait. Hence, a variety of situations have a common and uniquely individual significance to the person, and because these situations have a shared significance for the person which is somewhat different for other people, it tends to mediate a certain kind of behavior in common which is somewhat different from the behavior of other persons. He will behave in certain consistent ways, such as withdrawing, or perhaps, if the context is different, becoming overaggressive and domineering. This trait is actually nothing other than a class of meanings to a person of a variety of situations. Because these situations have a common meaning, the person behaves in predictable ways which are different from the way other people behave. This is how the problem of meaning comes into the center of personality.

The analysis in learning theory terms of the various types of psychodynamic mechanisms growing out of frustration and conflict also leads to the discovery of a meaningful or significant process central to all of them. Take, for example, a phobia. It is quite obvious that there is a central class of stimuli which have a unique and different significance or meaning for the phobic individual than for most people. In fact, the nature of the disturbed or deviant meanings is the definition of the type of phobic situation. The same sort of analysis can be made of each of the other psychodynamic mechanisms, of course. Projective techniques provide another example. Everyone agrees that when a clinician applies a relatively ambiguous stimulus to a subject — the Rorschach, TAT, or even a Szondi — he is interested in the types of responses the subject makes to it; he is quite literally studying the ways in which the meanings for this ambiguous stimulus are a function of the type of personality the subject has and the ways in which these meanings of significance vary from those of other people. Similarly in psychotherapy, one of the most important aspects of the behavior disorders is a disturbance in semantics — in the meaning of the self, the mother and father, the wife or husband, and other significant persons in the patient's life. One of the central phenomena of a person with a behavior disorder is thus a disturbance in the meaning system, and in the course of psychotherapy one of the essential things that happens is a change in the meaning system of the patient.

Most of the chapters in this book depict clinical and experimental approaches to the investigation of symbolism through the use of hypnotic technique. The value of hypnosis in dream research is that it apparently provides access to the symbol-translating mechanism. The process of symbolization has been at once one of the most intriguing and one of the most controversial aspects of the theory advanced by psychoanalysis. The major impediment to research in this field has been the extremely loose manner in which this theory has been formulated. In recognition of the need for a redefinition of terms and a statement of hypotheses

in testable form, this chapter will begin with an attempt to show
how the phenomenon of symbolization can be incorporated into
C. E. Osgood's mediation theory of behavior (1953).

A MEDIATION THEORY OF UNCONSCIOUS SYMBOLIZATION

The mediation theory was formulated for the express purpose of
providing a theoretical framework for research into the complex,
intervening process between stimulus and response in the human
organism. It originated from the premise that *meaning* is the central problem in contemporary psychology. According to this
theory, an object may elicit a complex pattern of reactions from
the organism, some of which are "object-tied" (depend upon the
sensory presence of the object for their occurrence) and others
which are "detachable" (can occur without presence of the object). Of the total pattern of detachable reactions conditioned by
the experience with the object, some fraction becomes the stable
mediation process (meaning) elicitable by various signs of the
object. In the human it is likely that these representational "reactions" become entirely central (neutral) in nature.

The development of meaning of a distal sign, for instance,
would be when, through manipulative experience with the object,
a small boy learns to respond to a toy gun by grasping the handle, pulling the trigger, and saying, "Bang! You're dead." According to the mediation theory, the visual patterns deriving from
the object will tend to become associated with some minimal but
distinctive portion of the total behavior which is the "perceptual
significance" or "meaning" of the visual pattern.

Verbal signs develop meaning in the same manner as do distal
perceptual cues. A sign is defined as "a pattern of stimulation
which is not the object, is a sign of the object when it elicits in
the organism a mediation process which (a) is some portion of
the same behavior made to the object and (b) mediates overt behavior which would not occur without previous association of the

sign and object patterns of stimulation" (Osgood, 1953). When
the sign-to-be is presented in conjunction with the object and/or
with the distal signs of the object, it tends to be conditioned to
the total reaction, but later, when the sign-to-be is presented
alone, only detachable reactions can be elicited. Early linguistic
signs typically acquire meaning through association with distal
stimuli; i.e., word meanings typically follow and depend on perceptual meanings. At later stages, more abstract linguistic signs
can acquire meaning via association with previously learned
signs, a process called "assign learning."

Freud differentiated between so-called "true symbols" and
other modes of indirect representation in dreams, such as substitution, allusion, and imagery. The "true symbol" was believed to
possess universal (usually sexual) meaning; i.e., "the relationship
between a symbol and the idea symbolized is an invariable one"
(Freud, 1953, p. 158), and therefore when encountered in a
dream, true symbols could be interpreted independently of the
dreamer's associations. The definition of a symbol as having a
constant, unconscious meaning is regarded as unnecessarily limited and is not subscribed to here. Freud himself admitted: "We
cannot at present assign quite definite limits to our conception of
a symbol; for it tends to merge into substitution, representation,
etc., and even approaches closely to allusion" (1953, p. 159).
There is no experimental evidence of the ability of hypnotic subjects to interpret dream symbolism generally; the evidence we do
have is that they are capable of translating their own symbols but
not the representations made by others.

The second criterion of the "true symbol" was that it represented unconscious content. Initially Freud maintained that censorship was the primary motive in dream distortion and the symbol was regarded simply as a means of disguise. As Jones stated,
". . . only what is repressed needs to be symbolized.
This . . . is the touchstone of the psychoanalytic theory of symbolism" (1950, p. 116). Later Freud recognized symbolism as
the natural expressive mode of dreams, but he continued to

maintain that symbolization serves the purpose of censorship by making the dream strange and incomprehensible. Practical and logical considerations indicate the desirability of a broadened definition to include all indirect modes of representation which issue from the transformation of latent into manifest dream content. This position does not seem incompatible with Freud's later formulation in which the mechanism of displacement was assigned a primary role in dream censorship. There are questions about the disguise function of symbolism which will be dealt with later.

As used here, *a symbol is simply a substitute for another idea from which, in the particular context such as a dream, it derives a secondary significance not inherent in itself.*

Both the linguistic sign and the symbol are related to the objects they represent by a similarity of mediational processes. However, while the sign is an arbitrary signifier, its relation to the object being established by social convention, the utilization of a symbol is typically a spontaneous event, dependent upon transfer through some intrinsic identity between two or more concepts. Thus the word "chair" is a conventional symbol, there being no inherent relationship between the phonemes or letters, or their arrangement, to the meaning of that which it signifies. In contrast, a fire possesses the qualities of movement, lightness, gaiety, and heat and therefore may symbolize a mood of aliveness and adventure. Shared experiences account for the generality of such symbols within a society or culture, but many symbols express a unique, autistic, personalized meaning. It is also characteristic of symbols that they are sensorial and concrete, whereas the idea represented may be relatively abstract and complex.

This is related to another distinction between sign and symbol — the former is characteristically employed in order to increase the precision of social thought and communication, while the motive for the symbol is usually the private expression of affect-laden content. There is one more distinction between the metaphor and the dream symbol. While the former is usually chosen to represent or accentuate one particular aspect, the latter is typically "overdetermined," that is, highly condensed, and therefore representative of several latent meanings. This factor of condensation may play a primary role in the fact that dreams are typically not understood by the waking subject.

In the mediation theory, the more similar the meaning of the content being symbolized to the ordinary meaning of the general concept to be used as a symbol, the more readily can the symbolization process occur. Given a drive for expression of the latent content, a shift in meaning from that associated with a symbol toward that associated with the latent content will occur more readily, the greater the degree of similarity among mediators. This is a straightforward instance of generalization among mediators. However, although increased semantic similarity enhances the possibility of symbolization, the resulting shifts in meaning must be less in magnitude. For example, if the specific mediator were a pencil, it could more easily become a symbol for a gun, a concept with which it shares a number of mediators, than it could for, say, a doll, an object which is semantically more distant. The shift of meaning in the process of symbolizing is obviously not as great.

A definite factor operative in the utilization of a symbol is the strength of motivation. Increased motivation toward expression of the latent content (i.e., the meaning of the object being symbolized) makes possible selection of more similar symbols. With a high drive, the person might actually dream of a potent expression of hostility toward a familiar person and perceive it as a nightmare. This derives from the fact that drive combines multiplicatively with habit strength to yield reaction potential. It should be noted that the drive strength affects both the amplitude of the mediational process characteristic of the object and the tendency to make the responses which this process mediates; i.e., the greater is the drive strength, the greater is the tendency to respond directly.

A discussion of the role of a competing drive, anxiety, is directly related to symbol choice in the question as to why symbolization is employed at all. Symbolization ostensibly occurs when a particular drive is present but not the mediating process ordinarily used to express it. When a dominant response is prevented from occurring, the next strongest may be expected to occur. When this substitution response is selected because of generalization among mediators, the process is called mediated generalization. In the present context this phenomenon will be called "displacement." In the simplest case, the young child's learned responses to a toy gun are inhibited by its absence. In the presence of a drive to express hostility, say, these responses may be expected to generalize to other similar objects, with stronger responses being elicited the more similar the new objects are in meaning to the original one. In this instance, the clenched fist and extended forefinger may be the most similar mediator readily available and the child will utilize it as a gun. While the total stimulus pattern may now elicit overt behavior appropriate to gun rather than to hand, it is presumed that the child retains awareness throughout that his gun is actually a hand and pointed finger. Thus, here there is identification only in terms of behavior and, hence, what may be termed conscious symbolism.

On the other hand, if under the impact of strong emotion the child were momentarily unaware that he had substituted a symbol, this would be called unconscious symbolism. The dream provides an example of the unconscious utilization of symbols; that is, in the dream there is usually no conscious recognition of employing a symbol, and the dreamer behaves toward it as he would the object. Use of the dream symbol would arise from (a) a drive toward expression of some affective content and (b) an aspect of similarity between the mediational processes of the symbol and of the affective content for which it substitutes. Because the symbol now elicits the mediational process characteristic of the thing being symbolized, there is not merely an identification in behavior (as with a conscious employment of a symbol) but a complete identification in meaning — hence what may be called unconscious symbolism. Between these extreme instances, of course, range all manner of intermediate stages. The distinction between conscious and unconscious symbolism remains relative — all thought, conscious from one angle, is unconscious from another. There is a continuous and fluid transition between consciousness and unconsciousness. In the most typical process of symbolization there is probably only a partial identification between the symbol and the content symbolized. For example, in the illustration a child uses his hand as a toy gun and to some degree he may retain awareness that he is utilizing the hand as a substitute. But in the heat of playing "cowboy," the hand also tends to elicit mediators characteristic of those developed in "gun" experiences, and his meaning is typically some compromise.

Freud, of course, attributed a disguise function to symbolism and postulated that a shift from one concept to another may occur due to the necessity of representing a prohibited desire in a disguised form. He conceptualized symbol selection as a compromise between two opposing forces, and the need to represent the covert thought stimulates anxiety. Perhaps without intention, psychoanalysts have often tended to reify the censorship force, making the mechanism and very existence of such a process difficult to grasp. Learning theorists would expect that when the direct response to the original stimulus is prevented by conflict, the inhibitory responses may be expected to generalize also. There is some experimental evidence that the inhibitory tendencies generalize less broadly (according to a sharper gradient) than excitatory tendencies. Apparently this is the mechanism responsible for the clinical phenomenon of displacement (Miller, 1944, 1948).

In terms of mediation theory, the latent content of a dream (e.g., the aggressive use of penis) may be represented as an impulse associated with its characteristic representational mediation process, while the manifest content or symbol (e.g., a pistol) is represented as a sign ordinarily associated with its own mediation process. Two basic drives are also postulated, the need for expression (motivation) and the need for avoidance (anxiety). In the conscious use of symbols, the drive for expression combines with the self-stimulation characteristic of the mediational processes of the symbol to modify overt behavior in the direction of that associated with the thing symbolized. But the meaning of the symbol as such is unaltered — for instance, a child using his forefinger as if it were a gun. Under the stress of emotion the child may temporarily lose his awareness of his hand. In the unconscious use of symbols, the mediation process characteristic of the symbol is shifted toward the meaning of the thing symbolized. For the dreamer, the symbol pistol acquires a meaning having some characteristics of penis as reflected in the acquisition of denotative qualities, such as a flexible barrel emitting a poisonous fluid rather than bullets, and so forth. Following is a dream reported by a 24-year-old woman, illustrating this shift:

> She was standing in the foyer of her home with her boyfriend. He pressed what appeared to be a wooden staff or stake into her hand. At first it was entirely inert, but then it began to writh and she was frightened that it was a snake and it might bite her. She frantically tried to call his attention to it, but he ignored her. Then her mother appeared and the boyfriend disappeared. Her mother attempted to get her to crush it beneath her heel; however, the girl managed to open the garden window and the snake disappeared.

There were a number of interpretations made by the woman to her dream, but she unhesitantly declared the snake represented her male friend's attempt to unfeelingly thrust his sex upon her.

This phenomenon may be further translated into the terms of the displacement mechanism. The strength of the drive toward commerce with the object itself has been indicated as one factor in symbol selection. Increasing the strength of the drive motivating expression of an impulse will raise the height of the whole gradient of generalization. Assuming the anxiety level to be constant, the point of displacement will shift in the direction of symbols that are more similar to the impulse seeking expression as drive toward expression is increased. Ordinarily, when there is no reason for disguise (low anxiety), symbols should be chosen on the basis of similarity, the most direct representation being selected.

Assuming that anxiety is a second factor operating in symbol selection, in conformance with the laws of generalization, the stronger the anxiety associated with a given stimulus, the wider the generalization of anxiety to similar objects. It is assumed that the greater the anxiety associated with an object, the more distant must be the symbol chosen to represent it, given a constant drive toward expression. Theoretically, if the inhibition is strong enough, not even remote symbolic responses will occur; i.e., the subject will wake up. Increasing the strength of the anxiety accompanying direct expression of a repressed impulse will shift the point of strongest displacement in the direction of symbols that are less similar to the impulse. In general, then, the greater the strength of the drive toward expression (anxiety being constant), the less remote will be the symbol chosen. Though selection would ordinarily be on the basis of mediational similarity, the greater the anxiety (expressive drive strength being constant), the more remote the symbol that will be chosen.

Psychoanalytic theory would predict that when anxiety is great, the symbols chosen should be semantically distant from the latent content, and when anxiety is low or absent, selected symbols should be relatively close. That is, to the extent that a symbol and the content represented are mediationally similar, the meaning of the symbol is transparent; when a symbol and the latent content are semantically distant, so that the waking mind has difficulty making the connection, the symbol may be said to be disguised. In contrast, the mediation theory of symbolism would predict *no difference* in the size of the distance measurements in the two conditions. In a sense, learning theory and psychoanalytic theory agree *under conditions where the two drives are varied independently* — but they usually are not. It is the intersection of two competing drives (to *express* and to *repress*) that is the key to the hypothesis. Anxiety resulting in prolonged frustration should cause an increasing drive for expression, the effect being to raise the gradient, counteract the effects of anxiety, and result in the selection of symbols that are semantically close to the latent content, that is, relatively at the same point as when anxiety is low. This is exactly the result obtained in the experiments by Moss (1961). These results suggest that symbolism constitutes a language of the sleeping mind, and will be employed regardless of whether the latent content stimulates anxiety. Very difficult methodological problems indicate the tentative nature of this conclusion, however.

If this is the case and dream symbols are not disguised, why doesn't the waking mind simply translate the symbols into their sign significance? Why are most dreams essentially meaningless? There appear to be at least five possible reasons.

1) Western man prides himself on maintaining a sharp distinction between the waking and dream worlds, and the American society in particular has always been irrevocably extratensive in temperament. Perhaps this strict demarcation is required by the difficult distinction that we feel forced to maintain between internal and external reality. Man might easily mistake his dreams for reality, were they not so clearly embedded in the familiar content of sleep; it is an undoubted convenience on awakening to be able to dismiss these discrepant experiences as purely illusionary.

2) The language of the sleeping mind is relatively unfamiliar to the waking mind. It is more or less metaphorical in nature, not unlike poetry; this is the dream's theatrical quality and there are relatively few adults who are at home with this type of expression. It taxes our waking logic to make inferences to the "covert content" represented by our nocturnal mediation.

3) It is also a rich type of poetry, if one may pursue the analogy a bit further. It is typically overdetermined, so that there is no simple one-to-one translation. Even a short dream is translatable into many times its original length. This is the factor of *condensation.* Freud wrote, "No other process contributes so much to concealing the meaning of a dream and to making the connec-

tion between the dream content and the dream thoughts recognizable" (1952, p. 52). And he was doubtless correct, but this is *not* the factor of symbol disguise.

4) Most dreams are not held in memory for very long — they fade in a moment or so. The best way of recalling a dream is *not to move the head* upon awakening, but most people do not have the time or the inclination to lie in bed pursuing the meaning of their dreams. It is the exceptional or unique or usually the last dream of the night that is held in memory even for a few scant seconds after awakening. The dreams we remember best are those which occur in the REM period just before we awaken, and because the electrophysiological evidence suggests that our dreams become progressively more complex as the night wears on, we are confronted by a dream that is infinitely more difficult to decipher than the pedestrian and mundane dreams that occur in earlier REM periods.

5) Finally, there is undoubtably much waking anxiety about the content of dreams; they often reflect the irrational motives underlying our behavior, and this makes the dreamer unresponsive to the interpretation of his sleeping mentation. Thus, the patient tends to react defensively about his dreams, but this anxiety is in retrospect rather than intruding itself into the dreams and working to establish the disguise of the symbols employed. As we shall see later, most dreams told by patients to their therapists are in part secondary elaborations, a construction rather than a reconstruction or pure projective material.

In the last analysis, from the viewpoint of psychotherapy it makes little difference whether or not dreams are actually disguised; the point is that whatever the reason, most people do not understand their dreams or even remember them, and are resistive to having them interpreted.

The ability of some hypnotic subjects to transform a suggested content into its symbolic equivalent has been used in an investigation of the process of cognitive interaction involved in meaning formation and change to which Osgood applies the principle of

congruity (pp. 76, 78). These changes never occur in isolation
from one another. Briefly, this principle states that whenever two
signs (or a sign and a symbol) are related by a linguistic copula
or an assertive reaction, the mediating reaction characteristic of
each shifts toward congruence with that of the other, the magnitude of the shift being inversely proportional to the original intensity of the two interacting reactions in isolation.

In dream symbol formation, a situation obtains in which the
interaction of two signs is momentarily complete; that is, the
meaning of each sign is completely shifted to a point of mutual
congruence. The latent content is never trivial, since it has powerful affective and cognitive processes associated with it; in contrast, the manifest content has a preference for recent impres-
sions usually of an innocuous or affectively indifferent nature.
Therefore, the affect investing the latent content is always more
intense than is present in the manifest content, and the flow of
significance is invariably from the primary idea to the secondary
sign or symbol. The affect accompanying the dream is always appropriate to the latent content. At this moment there is a total
credulity on the part of the experiencing subject and he accepts
the symbol as reality.

And yet dreaming supposedly has a cathartic effect, for example, *reducing* anxieties, and if this is true, why does it happen
behaviorally? If this complete shift to meaning of the latent content is true, then there is good reason why the remoteness of a
symbol makes absolutely no difference in affect discharge, despite the problem of why it is not recognized as being the object
which it actually represents. The important thing here is the distinction between *affective* and other components of meaning; in
effect, dreams serve to infuse denotative signs, say, neckties, with
affective meaning, appropriate to penis. Perhaps, then, we have a
motivational conflict (expression vs. anxiety) determining *content* of dreams (symbol selection) and *cognitive interaction*
(affective and denotative features fusing as in phrases like "this
necktie is a penis") determining the *meaning* of the dream. Note

that the dream symbol has the affective features of the latent content and the nonaffective features of the manifest content.

As the relation diverges from perfect simultaneity between the two mediational processes, however, the magnitude of the congruity effect decreases, perhaps as a negatively accelerated function of time. A process of decoding usually occurs. The effect of one sign upon another decreases as the time interval between them increases, particularly when the subject awakens and the usual time-space logic resumes. Only upon awakening does the dreamer recognize, in retrospect, that his symbols were not reality, but he often does not recognize that they were also an allegorical expression of some underlying content. The exception to this rule occurs if, when the dreamer is highly motivated to continue the identity of the two signs even though he is awake, he is then confronted with a so-called neurotic and even psychotic distortion. Take, for example, the paradigm in which the subject was caught up in a bind of fearing pregnancy or losing her boyfriend: on the basis of a prior reaction (the detumescent penis looked like a shrunken hotdog) she apparently developed a phobic fear of hotdogs which was revealed in nightmares and real life without recapturing the response which was its basis.

In a concrete example, the interaction between the concept to be influenced, NEGRO, and the source of the influence, HYPNOTIST, was conceptualized within the model provided by the principle of congruity (see Chapter Five). With respect to EXPERIMENTER (hypnotist), while the attitudes of the control group became less favorable because of the nature of his communication, the attitudes of the experimental group became slightly more favorable. These predictions generated by the congruity principle held up well with respect to the direction of attitude change, although the magnitude of the changes for both groups was small. A question was raised as to whether the obtained original ratings of NEGRO were as negative as the subjects' "true" feelings. Nevertheless, this was a well-controlled, objective test of the congruity principle, which seems to show that a single application of a positive communication delivered under hypnosis about a current, sensitive topic is persuasive. The experimenters hesitated to follow up with added hypnotic inducements favoring this change because of the possibility they might be accused of "brainwashing" the subjects.

Coming back to the study of the disguise function of dream symbolism, despite difficult methodological problems, the results tend to be substantiated by an analysis of the principle of congruity. Let us say that the latent content is penis and the overt symbolism is, say, a metal stove poker. When the anxiety about the covert content is very high and the person has selected this particular symbol, then the dream-work according to Freud should function to make the characteristics of the manifest symbol less like (to distort or disguise) the underlying content; on the other hand, when the anxiety is reduced so there is little concern associated with the thing being symbolized, then the symbol should become semantically more like the covert content. The poker in this instance should become red rather than black, somewhat flexible rather than rigid, warm rather than cold, and so on — all of which is movement toward the thing being symbolized.

If associative assertion is true in dreams as it is in waking word mixtures, the learning theory analysis or congruity principle would posit that the movement of the symbol must always be toward the meaning of the highly affective underlying content and this is exactly what the author found. The meaning of the dream symbols was always away from the meaning of the symbol per se and the dream-work never resulted in additional features being added to the symbol to further disguise it; instead, the direction of the change in meaning was always toward the meaning of the latent content, regardless of the degree of anxiety associated with the covert content.

The research of Osgood and his associates (Osgood, 1964) over the past few years provides evidence for a universal framework underlying certain affective or connotative aspects of language. These findings increase the possibility of constructing instruments for measuring these aspects of "subjective culture" comparably in diverse societies — in effect, circumventing the language barrier. Beginning in 1960 these investigators sought to apply a design which would rigorously test the limits of possible generality for measuring similarities and differences in certain aspects of subjective culture — the affective or emotive aspects. To date they have studied some 25 language-culture groups. The major hypothesis that human beings share a common framework for differentiating the affective meaning of signs has been clearly borne out in the data. The dominant factors in the affective meaning system are evaluation, potency, and activity, usually in that order. Some differences between language-culture communities are, of course, found. In their future work the investigators plan to apply a short-form differential derived from the pan-cultural factor analysis to the development that might be called a "World Atlas of Affective Meanings." This will involve a greatly expanded set of concepts, deliberately selected for their intercultural discriminating power.

Theoretically, a variation of this system could be found to hold for the most subjective language of all, the language of dreams. The language of the sleeping mind, at least in Stage 1–REM, is in a very real sense a foreign language for the waking mind of all cultures. Very little of it is understandable even though each person spends two to three hours every night producing this type of mentation. Fromm (1951) posits that the foreignness and distortion in dreams are attributable to the mode of thought that obtains in the state of sleep consciousness. He emphasizes that symbolism is the only language common to all races and ages, and as such its study should be included in the curriculum of institutions of higher learning: "I believe that symbolic language is the one foreign language that each of us must learn. Its understanding brings us in touch with one of the most significant sources of wisdom, that of the myth, and it brings us in touch with the deeper layers of our own personality" (p. 10).

The highly generalized nature of the affective reaction system — the fact that it is independent of any particular sensory modality and yet participates with all of them — appears to be the psychological basis for the universality of the three factors of shared affective responses. Osgood states that the generalized nature of the emotive reaction system appears because "such diverse sensory experiences as a *white* circle (rather than black), and a *straight* line (rather than crooked), a *rising* melody (rather than a falling one), a *sweet* taste (rather than a sour one), a *caressing* touch (rather than an irritating scratch) can all share a common affective meaning that one can easily and lawfully translate from one modality into another in synesthesia and metaphor" (1964, p. 199).

In this article, Osgood also reports that it is now abundantly clear that the semantic differential technique taps only one, restricted aspect of meaning. Another important aspect of meaning is what can be called *denotative meaning*. By "denotative" he refers to the descriptive use of signs as contrasted with their emotive use. He writes:

> The problem comes out clearly in the verbal-behavior laboratory when we try to account fully for the phenomena of mediated (or semantic) generalization; associative bonds between training and test words account for a part of the variance and affective or connotative similarity as indexed by the semantic differential for another part, but there is still a large chunk of variance unaccounted for, and it presumably is that due to what we are calling denotative similarity. An adequate measure should reflect the multi-dimensional nature of meaning, should yield a quantitative measure of degrees of denotative similarity, should be completely general for all pairs of terms measured, and should meet the usual criteria of reliability, validity, and comparability across subjects and concepts (p. 198).

He concludes that "The development of a satisfactory quantitative measure of denotative meaning appears to me to be one of the most important problems for contemporary psycholinguistics."

This again brings us back to one major methodological impediment to the measurement of the effect of anxiety on the dream censorship process. It appears to be the consensus that dream symbols accurately portray the connotative meaning of the covert content. There is a flow of affective significance from the covert sign to the secondary symbol. Where the distortion (or disguise) takes place is in the denotative aspects of the symbol. This limitation of the semantic differential was recognized in the early investigation of the problem of the disguise function of dream symbols (Moss, 1960c), and while an attempt was made to devise a denotative differential at that time, obviously the efforts were only preliminary. The semantic differential clearly fails to reflect denotative similarities in any consistent fashion. The general hypothesis is that if a series of concepts, falling into different implicit classes (say, BABY vs. SPIKE), are judged comparatively on single semantic differential scales one at a time, the scales will tend to be used denotatively to the extent that they have denotative properties. Osgood (1964) states, "By assessing the dimensionality of the scale-space under these conditions we may be able to generate a denotative semantic space. Such a space will certainly contain many more factors than the affective semantic space" (p. 198).

The point is that the use of hypnosis in conjunction with the semantic differential, conceived within the mediation theory of behavior, seems to hold great promise for capturing in measurable form this mercurial interaction between representational processes which involves the acquisition and modification of sign significance involved in the process of symbolization. The eventual development of a denotative differential will go a long way toward clarifying the precise relationship between sign and symbol.

PART II   CLINICAL STUDIES

EIGHT

Representative Case Studies

I. A CASE OF WAR NEUROSIS [1]

The patient, aged 32, with an I.Q. of 103, service-connected for a chronic anxiety reaction, reported a consistent pattern of neurotic behavior since the torpedoing of his ship in 1943 when only two out of 101 men in his compartment survived. He enlisted at the age of 17 following completion of tenth grade and he reportedly had only five days of training at "bootcamp" (he didn't even know how to swim when he was sent to sea). He was in six major naval engagements in the ensuing eleven months. At the time his ship was torpedoed, he was three decks below the waterline, serving as an ammunition carrier. The lights immediately went out and fire engulfed the ship. The patient fought his way to a ladder and after a seemingly interminable period of time, he emerged on deck. He recalls being struck at the time by perceiving that he had two sets of hands — his own and a second set of burned flesh that hung down, resembling the shape of his hands. Ironically, a photograph of the patient swathed in bandages appeared in a national magazine and later was used as a Navy enlistment poster. Since that episode, any stimuli faintly reminiscent of combat, such as violence on television or even a thunderstorm, stimulated

[1] Much of this material is derived from the article, "Therapeutic Suggestion and Autosuggestion," reprinted by permission of *Journal of Clinical and Experimental Hypnosis*, 4, no. 2 (April, 1958): 109–115.

nightmares in which he relived the experience, leaving him tense, highly irritable, withdrawn (as a defense against his rage reactions), and unable to work.

The patient had received professional assistance for the past 12 years without appreciable relief. He tried first for a position with a professional baseball team but failed, and then he attempted to become an umpire, but he became very angry whenever his calls were challenged. Finally, he obtained his present position as a glass beveler, and fortunately his employers were very permissive and tolerated the patient's nervousness and his frequent absences. The present treatment problem was complicated by his generalized claustrophobia, including an intense fear of hospital confinement, and pressing financial obligations. He promised to stay only three weeks and the problem was to develop a brief, effective treatment program. Hypnosis seemed the method of choice.

A basic question concerned the reason for the ego's failure to assimilate or repress the traumatic experience. This was in effect the retroactive mastery of stress which Freud emphasized, i.e., the repeated attempts of the patient to gain mastery of a traumatic experience that has overwhelmed him. It was originally hypothesized that in his life-and-death struggle, the patient might have committed some action resulting in unresolved repressed guilt. Hypnosis was used to revivify the original trauma. As a precaution, the emotional involvement was initially controlled by having the patient view the event on an imaginary movie screen. An important variation in technique involved time-distortion; the scenes were to be "played" in slow motion, allowing control of affective responses and also minute examination of an action which had actually occurred in approximately 90 seconds. Although memory for the event was clarified, no important new dynamic elements were disclosed. It was concluded that this trauma had been experienced as a crushing defeat for an already insecure ego and had exaggerated a basically passive-dependent adjustment.

Thereafter several supportive hypnotic techniques were employed, designed to alleviate the patient's severe incapacitation. It was considered of primary importance to control the disrupting effect of his nightmares. It was discovered that dreams occurred with greater frequency when the patient slept on his back, so it was suggested under hypnosis that he not sleep on his back and that his unconscious prevent him from rolling over. A second hypnotic suggestion was that whenever such a dream began he would immediately awaken. These dreams were conceptualized as the ego's attempt to assimilate the trauma and therefore completely halting them could have a deleterious effect. A secondary controlled mode of expression was allowed through continued employment of the movie screen technique, accompanied by the repeated suggestion that the ego discriminate past and present experiences.

Hypnotic suggestions of relaxation and support were also employed as a sedative during periods of excessive tension. According to the patient's report the effects of these suggestions continued for three or four days and thereafter progressively diminished. It was recognized that a large part of his immediate, dramatic improvement was attributable to satisfaction of his strong dependency needs. In order to modify this relationship, beginning in the third month the patient was trained in autohypnosis. He was taught, for instance, to relax himself whenever he felt particularly tense or irritable. He learned to counteract a tendency toward insomnia by the same technique. As he gained in self-comfort, he was encouraged to examine the basis for his interpersonal difficulties and to attempt a realistic solution. Increased self-control apparently resulted in a general gain in self-confidence.

Appointments were left to the patient's own discretion. He was seen for 12 sessions before being discharged, returned once a week for two months, and thereafter averaged one "maintenance" visit per month for the next year, when the relationship was terminated. Although the patient's basic personality pattern was unaltered, his symptoms were less troublesome and his general adjustment improved.

A vignette taken from the fifteenth session is more or less typical of the interaction with this patient.

P: I was driving down the highway — it was just out of Toledo. It was raining real hard, and I could barely see. It was funny, I could just about see the ornament on the hood of the car. I wanted to pull over to the side, but I was afraid of getting stuck in the mud, so I slowed down, and it was then that the bolt of lightning hit. It was just straight streaks, straight down and it just burst. And everything disappeared, and I don't know how far in front of us but it wasn't too far. And then it seemed like the rain cleared, and when we got up in front of us, the lightning had hit this tree. Just right after it hit was when I started feeling a funny feeling in my chest and my stomach, and one hand started to shake a bit. Then I drove into a little town on up there, and my dad drove the rest of the way.

T: Can you tell me a little more in detail how you felt after that lightning hit?

P: Well, I wanted to stop the car right then and get out of the car, but like I say, it was raining a little bit and there was nothing else I could do, so I just drove the car to this little town. That's when we changed driving; I asked him if he would drive the rest of the way, and I just sat in the front seat. Before that hit, we had gone through other rains and lightning and it wasn't too bad, but just as soon as that hit, then I just felt like I was through with the trip right there.

T: It shook you up that much?

P: Uh huh. I didn't tell him that, but he knew something was wrong.

T: Well, how long afterwards did it continue to affect you?

P: We were going to stay up in Toledo with this fellow, and I couldn't sit still. I'd sit down awhile and read a book, and it happened to be right on the lake front, and I went down to the lake front and watched some ore ships, watched them load and unload coal, and then I'd come back in and sit down awhile. We were up there for two days.

T: You were restless all this time?

P: The whole time.

T: You think this has something to do with this bolt of lightning?

P: I know that. I mean I felt pretty good about going up there until it hit, and then I didn't care anymore.

T: How long ago was that now?

P: Well, I can't remember the date, but I read in the paper the same day that you people down here had a terrific storm that blew over the Jubilee thing because it was in the paper up there. They had a picture of it.

T: That was several weeks ago. And you haven't been able to pull yourself together since then?

P: Well, it's like I said, I've noticed myself a little crabby at work and at home and I've been just driving around in my car at night, just unable to settle down.

T: What do you think happened to you in that instant?

P: Well, I mean it was so clear, I had seen it before, something like that.

T: It was as if you had been through this thing before?

P: It was just as clear as a bell, this burst when it hit the tree trunk, it was just like a ball of fire. That's all there was to it.

T: *Have* you been through this before?

P: Well, I can remember in the service, the bomb hits and this is the way they acted. Only with them there was smoke that followed them, but this one, there was just one flash and it was all over with.

T: So, for just a second, you were back in your combat experience again?

P: Well, I would say after watching the ball of fire, there was something that made me feel that way. Now, if I had stopped and listened to my dad's advice and not gone on, I don't know what would have happened. If we had stopped in this spot, maybe the bolt, we'd have never seen it. Maybe I would have been five or 10 miles away from it, more than we actually were.

T: Does this make you feel that you should have listened to your father?

P: Well, I feel after it was all over that it was unnecessary to drive that extra distance.

T: Why do you think this one, short, split-second episode should upset you so much?

P: Well, like I say, when something like that happens, I start to thinking about when I was in the Navy. This little episode that flashed back and forth in front of me. I can do it sitting at home or at work, anywhere. And like I said before, I don't want to read it in the papers or hear it on television, or anything like that.

T: You'd like to completely avoid it if you can?

P: I'd like to, yes.

T: So even after all these 12 years, something like that will call back what you went through in the Navy and get you disturbed for several days or a week?

P: It seems like anything that's fire or water, like thunder or rain or even fire. I don't like them.

T: Do you think that you will ever be able to get over these experiences, these memories? Or do you think they will always come back to haunt you when you have an experience such as you describe?

P: I don't know what will happen. I'm doing all right, day by day, it's a good day and I'm feeling pretty good. But when the clouds start to cloud up, and everything seems like it's closing in on me, that's when I feel a little restless, like this thunderstorm, like that, I get a little restless.

T: You feel as though you were being trapped in a situation over which you have no control?

P: Well, I just feel like everything is closing in on me, and I have to find some way to get out.

T: Some way to escape?

P: Well, as I told you before, during a storm at night, I wake up and go to the front door and look at the windows so that I know there is some way to get out of there if something happens which, so far outside of being scared of the lightning, nothing much else has happened.

T: But in spite of the fact that your fears are groundless and it has been shown to you again and again, it still upsets you, doesn't it?

P: Yes, it does.

T: Why don't you sit back and relax? I'll help you to relax with a few suggestions and perhaps I can help you get into this episode in a little more detail. Do you want to do that?

P: Last time I left here, it was a week or two weeks, I got a lot of rest, so it seemed like from leaving here, I got a lot of rest.

T: You get something out of these sessions which helps you to relax?

P: When I left here and went home, I laid down and slept a pretty good length of time.

[Hypnosis induced.]

T: Now we're going back in time, back to a couple of weeks ago, back to when you were driving down the road going to Toledo, going to Toledo with your father. You are driving down the road, it's raining, and it is getting harder all the time. The rain is falling harder all the time; tell me what is going on.

P: The rain comes down over the window, we close up the car. It's hot in here, no ventilation, can't see nothing, it's hot.

T: It's hot and close in here, isn't it?

P: Yes. I'm scared. Scared and don't want to stop, want to keep moving. I want to get out of there. Dad's talking to me, a big flash, right in front of the car, a ball of fire, disappears. I'm scared, start to shake, notice my hands shaking. I almost stop the car.

T: Now, I want you to go back in time, back to another situation, an earlier time when you felt the same way. The picture is forming, you're beginning to see it clearly. Describe to me where you are.

P: I'm standing on a ship. The ship I'm on is a garbage grinder. I couldn't get down to my battle station. I stood by the garbage grinder and watched the planes attack this ship. One dove right down and I couldn't see anything but a ball of fire. It started smoking. Gotta get out of here, get back in behind the door. I closed the door. I'm scared.

T: What are you feeling and thinking during this time?

P: I'm scared, wondering if it's gonna hit us.

T: You're afraid that you're going to be killed?

P: Yes.

T: How about your hands?

P: Shaking all over.

T: Now listen to my voice. You are coming back through time. You will recall the experience you just told me, you can see now that this bolt of lightning made you remember a very vivid experience while you were in combat, an experience in which you were afraid of being killed. But you must keep this in mind; as terrible as the experiences you had in service were, they are behind you, they are in the past. Every once in a while, you get into a situation now which reminds you of the past. There is something similar about it, like that bolt of lightning reminds you of the ball of fire that the plane made coming down on the ship. But you know consciously and unconsciously that these are not the same situations, the bolt of lightning reminds you of a terrible experience in the past. But it is past, you must accept the past. It is gone and it will never come again. You must make a clear distinction. The only reality to the past is in terms of your feelings about it. You must not confuse the past with the present. Its only reality is in your feelings. And your feelings are not always fact, sometimes your feelings lie to you.

[Patient was allowed to remain in hypnosis for several additional minutes in which positive suggestions were given concerning his well being, his ability to rest and relax, and his ability to control reaction to stimuli which formerly upset him. Patient then awakens.]

T: How do you feel?

P: Good.

T: What's going through your mind?

P: I was thinking about that bolt of lightning I was talking to you about. It was the same as when I was on the ship, the end of it, the fire was the same. Almost alike. I saw a plane drop a bomb on a carrier one time, I saw a red ball of fire out there; he let it go and pulled out of his dive.

T: So apparently this bolt of lightning brought back the memory of this instance?

P: Well, that's what I think of.

T: Do you think that's what happened to you on the road when this bolt of lightning hit — it transported you back?

P: I know I felt funny and I had to get out of there.

T: We've talked about this before and I think this is one more example of how the experiences you went through in service cause you today to be sensitive to anything that reminds you of them. I think you can see here how momentarily you confused the past and the present.

P: That's what the ball of fire made me think of. One looked almost identical to the other one.

T: Do you think that you've made much progress in getting over your combat experiences? Do they bother you as much as they used to, say, before we began these sessions?

P: Well, if I get down here and talk to you before I stay away too long; I can feel myself get to a point of where I don't even want to read about it in the newspaper. I want to throw it all aside, I don't want to hear it or see it. I don't want to hear anything about it, I don't want to see it in the movies or anything like that. And then when I start noticing myself starting to snap at everybody at home and at work, well then I try to get in touch with you. It seems like I'm a whole lot better after I leave here for a length of time until there is anything that starts it all over again.

In this study, the semantic differential was employed for the objective measurement of the feeling aspects of meaning. Table 10 reports a comparison of the *distance measures* of the ratings of 15 concepts made by the patient at the beginning, middle, and end of treatment.

TABLE 10. Quantitative changes in the meaning of 15 concepts at three stages in psychotherapy.

Concept	Ratings		
	I-II	II-III	I-III
ACTUAL SELF	9.80	6.56	11.09
IDEAL SELF	2.24	2.00	1.73
WIFE	13.08	1.73	13.15
CHILDREN	3.16	1.73	3.00
MOTHER	6.16	6.71	2.83
FATHER	5.57	6.25	2.45
PEOPLE	13.71	6.48	12.33
COMBAT EXPERIENCE	1.73	1.73	.00
NIGHTMARES	5.19	3.79	6.16
MY ILLNESS	3.16	6.63	6.08
JOB	8.37	2.45	7.48
SENSE OF FAILURE	2.83	7.21	8.25
THERAPY	13.96	5.38	15.56
HYPNOSIS	8.37	2.00	8.83
THERAPIST	8.83	2.24	8.54

Note: Figures were obtained by squaring the difference on each of 13 scales, summing, and taking the square root. The larger is the number, the greater the difference, the smaller the number, the less the difference.

Qualitative analysis of the ratings provides considerable information regarding changes in meaning experienced by the patient during psychotherapy. Perception of the ACTUAL SELF concept changed markedly throughout treatment, while there were only chance fluctuations in ratings of the IDEAL SELF concept. These results are consistent with numerous studies which find the IDEAL SELF concept highly stable. The stability of this concept over a 15-month period provides a measure of reliability of repeated measurements of a single concept when no alterations in meaning occur. A contrast of the ratings of the ACTUAL and IDEAL SELF

concepts obtained at each rating also reveals a progressive decrease in the semantic distance and suggests an increasing degree
of self-acceptance. These results are again consistent with
changes reported in the literature. Also consistent with this interpretation is the decrease in the patient's sense of personal failure.

Five of the concepts reflect the patient's interpersonal relationships. A considerable initial alienation toward the wife is greatly
reduced. The patient's children are regarded in a uniformly positive fashion and there are no gross qualitative changes in attitude
toward the parents. However, the patient's attitude toward people
in general undergoes considerable change in a more positive
direction. A somewhat increased satisfaction with his job also
reflects an improved relationship with fellow-workers with whom
he had previously feuded.

The patient's memory of his combat experiences shows no evidence of desensitization (and perhaps it should not). Nevertheless, the negative connotation of both his nightmares and his
illness is quantitatively reduced. The three related concepts measuring the patient's attitude toward psychotherapy (THERAPY,
THERAPIST, and HYPNOSIS) indicate an increasingly favorable
attitude.

While over-all changes are represented in Table 10, the scales
purport to measure three different aspects of meaning, and results
can be analyzed on this basis. The greatest change occurred between Ratings I and II and the largest proportion of this was on
Factor I, the evaluation dimension. Represented by seven scales,
four of these (happy-sad, valuable-worthless, kind-cruel, and
good-bad) are much more sensitive to change than the remaining
three (sweet-sour, ugly-beautiful, dirty-clean). Changes in meaning between Ratings II and III were more highly influenced by
alterations on the remaining potency and activity factors with the
largest contribution being made by a general reversal of ratings
on the hot-cold scale (activity dimension). Inquiry elicited that
the patient associated "heat" with his claustrophobia reaction so

that this scale may be interpreted as reflecting feelings of anxiety or discomfort for the patient.

A final analysis concerned which units of the seven-point scales the patient used in making his ratings. The manner in which patients use the differential has suggested that the units checked may have some individual (possibly diagnostic) significance. Predominant use of the extreme units (1 and 7) reflects judgment in terms of opposites, a black-white type of reasoning. Theoretically, improvement with psychotherapy should result in greater discrimination as indicated by a broader use of the scale units. Unfortunately for the hypothesis (and the patient), he used the same units with considerable uniformity throughout; the patient made negligible use of the middle (neutral) category, used the 1-7 categories predominantly, and used the 2-6 and 3-5 units with decreasing frequency.

A frequently expressed objection to the use of hypnosis in psychotherapy is that such treatment is purely symptomatic and temporary; this appears to be much less of an obstacle than it was before behavior therapy came into vogue. The thesis proposed here is that symptomatic relief is a legitimate therapeutic goal and that skillfully applied hypnosis provides a method of greatly increasing suggestive potency. The patient stated that he felt "better than at any time in years." On the other hand, it was recognized that these methods were limited in their objectives, but they were designed to begin helping the patient to assimilate his trauma, control his anxiety-dominated reactions, and start to adjust on a more realistic level. It was, in effect, a first step toward eventual rehabilitation. The effective factors in treatment seem to have been (a) the substitution of an active for a passive experience via hypnosis, (b) re-experiencing the trauma in as large a dose as the subject could manage, giving rise to the discharge of pent up tension, and (c) cognitive insight. Insight is beneficially complemented throughout by a reconditioning procedure and thus therapy is shortened to a much greater extent, without any attempt to alter the basically passive-dependent character of the patient.

II. THE CASE OF ALICE M.[2]

The patient, aged 31, Catholic, a divorcee, and mother of three daughters (ages 11-17), was a voluntary hospital admission, diagnosed psychoneurotic reaction, conversion type. Her main complaints were of periodic feelings of unreality and "seizures," both of about six months' duration. These convulsive episodes were typically brief; she was said to scream and thrash about on the floor and to claim amnesia for them. She had one previous hospitalization, five months earlier, staying only two weeks when her symptoms disappeared.

Individual psychotherapy was recommended and she was referred to a female staff psychologist. After 10 sessions the therapist asked for a consultation with the author. She related that Alice remained anxious, restless, and complaining, and had recently manifested a major seizure during staff ward rounds. She also relayed the patient's request that hypnosis be employed in order to expedite treatment. The highlights of these first 10 sessions are summarized as follows.

1) Alice frequently complained of feelings of unreality, as expressed in the verbalization, "Nothing seems real around me. Even I don't feel real. It's like I'm running away from something and don't know what it is."

2) She often revealed an autonomy-dependency conflict. While strongly resentful of treatment as an irresponsible child by people, she expressed frank fear of adult responsibilities. A seeming consequence was recurrent depressive episodes, in which she characterized herself as feeling "like a small child, like a nothing."

3) Alice identified sex as a major problem. She stated, "I was

[2] Reprinted by permission of the *Journal of Clinical and Experimental Hypnosis*, 10 (1962): 59–74.

a wife to my husband in every way except sexually — I couldn't stand to have him touch me." She recalled that while her mother reputedly despised men and rejected sex, she had frequent extra-marital affairs. Alice reported having always felt closer to her father and even having "double-dated" with him as a young teen-ager, though she also recounted a vague impression that as a lit-tle girl "he did something that frightened me." There was recall that at age six she had to repulse sexual advances by an older brother.

4) The patient also acknowledged that her relationship with her oldest daughter, Connie, constituted a considerable problem. She described Connie as resentful and rebellious. "I was always trying to win her love and never could. No matter what I'd do, it was never enough, she never showed any appreciation. I always tried so hard to give my girls what I never had."

While the preliminary sessions had been productive, it seemed likely that hypnosis could facilitate treatment. Alice proved to be a rather petite and attractive blond, quite feminine in a rather girlish manner. The initial impression was of an immature, unsta-ble, and passive-dependent personality. She was a moderately ca-pable hypnotic subject. It was agreed to see her once a week and to employ hypnosis as a catalyst in the rapid uncovery of re-pressed content, while her primary therapist would continue a conventional therapy relationship on a three-times-per-week basis. The patient readily accepted this restructuring.

Intensive, long-term psychotherapy, designed to effect a per-sonality reconstruction and directed at the goal of independent self-management, seemed completely unrealistic, and a more modest plan was agreed upon by the two therapists. For a year Alice had been caught in a dilemma composed of two men, her ex-husband, Frank, and a lover. Frank had been a competent provider but she had hated sexual relations with him; the second man made her feel "loved" and she enjoyed physical contact with him, but he was irresponsible and had been unable to make her feel materially secure. Material considerations were of special importance because Alice wanted the three daughters with her. It was decided to focus on the psychological barriers which might prevent Alice from re-establishing a comfortable dependency in a marriage relationship.

An obvious item meriting scrutiny was Alice's Catholicism; however, this did not seem to occasion her much concern. She did state that her conversion to Catholicism five years earlier was attributable to a lifelong fear of death, and volunteered a recurrent, extremely realistic, and terrifying childhood dream, which was in some inexplicable fashion related to this fear. It was decided to use this dream as the initial entree into an exploration of the patient's problems.

Dream. She walked into her bedroom and there in the dark stood a small, furry, white dog. Though it tried to be friendly and snuggle up to her, she was very frightened. She edged out of the bedroom and when the dog tried to follow, she managed to close the door. [The dream would invariably awaken her and she would sleep the remainder of the night on the living room sofa.]

Hypnoanalysis of the dream yielded a seemingly clear example of the disguise function of dream symbolism in a young child. The effort was first made to help Alice decipher the symbol using a familiar movie screen translation technique (Moss, 1960c, 1961); however, the mere perception of the "puppy" even after 23 years still occasioned her great terror. A secondary method designed to increase emotional distance and also to allow a more public representation of the symbol was instituted. In hypnosis Alice was handed a pencil and paper and told that when she opened her eyes, she would "see" the dog in her dream clearly etched on the paper and that she was to trace carefully over this outline. After successfully complying with these instructions, she was then told that when she opened her eyes again, she would see an outline of an image representing the central meaning of the little dog and she was to again "trace these lines exactly as they appear there on the paper" (see Fig. 8).

Upon completion, Alice suddenly recognized the full significance of the drawings and abreacted strongly. She identified the second drawing as her grandfather in his coffin and the little white dog as a symbol of death. She recalled that as a very small girl she and the grandfather had close, affectionate ties, but that he died when she was six. However, she did not fully comprehend the meaning of his death, and her parents had told her he was "sleeping." When she was eight she observed the dead body of a neighbor woman's baby, and suddenly, for the first time, she experienced the full emotional impact of the loss of the beloved grandfather. That night she had the disturbing nightmare. To date she had been obsessed by the need to touch dead bodies, as if striving for some explanation of death in this manner.

Asked the significance of the dog, she replied, "Death is cold, black, ugly. It was a pretty, little white dog, but I was afraid of it. It wasn't large, black, or cold; it was warm, cuddly, and white. I think I must have rejected the idea of death and put something else in its place, something pretty and nice, something that wasn't horrible."

An investigation of Alice's "feelings of unreality" led to the next major therapeutic development. These feelings antedated hospitalization by several months and were vaguely related to her

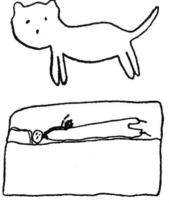

FIG. 8. Projected desymbolization of a dream symbol.

seizures, which began about the same time. She began the session with a reference to the recent seizure experienced during ward rounds. "I got terribly upset," she recalled, "though I don't know why. I had told Dr. A. that I was ready to go home to my sister's and go to work, and he told me he had written to get her. I got awfully afraid and just went to pieces. And afterwards, for one whole day, I thought I was a Joan Whitmier. The thought scared me, 'cause I thought, supposing I wouldn't know my mother when she came, or the members of my family? It scared me so I pushed it out of my mind. I kept telling myself, 'No, I'm Alice M.' I was afraid if I didn't convince myself that I would become this Joan Whitmier and maybe stay her." Thus Alice revealed for the first time the presence of an embryonic second personality.

Through hypnosis direct contact with Joan was readily established, allowing a detailed characterization and comparison with the conscious, dominant personality. Joan described herself as the same age as Alice but single, without children, and interested only in drinking, dancing, dating, nice clothes, and so forth. She was also fully conversant with Alice and her current difficulties. A most evident contrast was that Joan wanted absolutely no responsibilities. She explained that she came into existence as a consequence of Alice's extreme ambivalence about leaving the hospital and pursuing an independent existence. "Alice likes to be a strong and good person and shoulder the responsibility of her children, and be a good mother to them, and take good care of them. She wants to set a good example in front of them, that they can live by, and grow up to be good girls. Yet, every now and then when she tries to do these things, I come along and keep her from it."

In an effort to achieve additional insight into the nature and existence of Joan, the technique of automatic writing was introduced with partial success. Joan first printed her name, drew her self-portrait, and when asked for further clarification, repetitively reproduced two symbolic designs (Fig. 9). Analysis through a series of suggested drawings of increasing transparency of meaning led to the impression that the first design represented a preoccupation with sex (the outline depicted the head of a man Alice had intended to marry as a young girl but who had rejected her, and the internal lines represented sexual congress), while the second drawing symbolized Alice's feelings of confinement and frustration in an unmanageable marriage relationship. Later in the waking state, Alice immediately identified Joan's self-portrait (from the hair style) as herself when she was about 14. She recalled and was distressed by the conversation with Joan but seemed to accept an interpretation in terms of the conflict and dissociation of incompatible infantile and adult motives. Alice never again mentioned the existence of Joan, and the therapist felt it was strategic to avoid encouraging this dissociative tendency through further exploration. Semantic differential profiles obtained from Joan and contrasting ratings of Joan and Alice are of interest (D = 15.20) (Fig. 10).

A third significant therapeutic advance was achieved three weeks later when the patient recalled her unhappy childhood and her intense jealousy of a younger sister whom she felt had de-

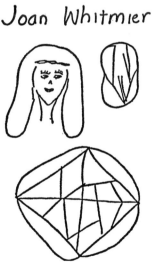

FIG. 9. Automatic drawings of a secondary personality.

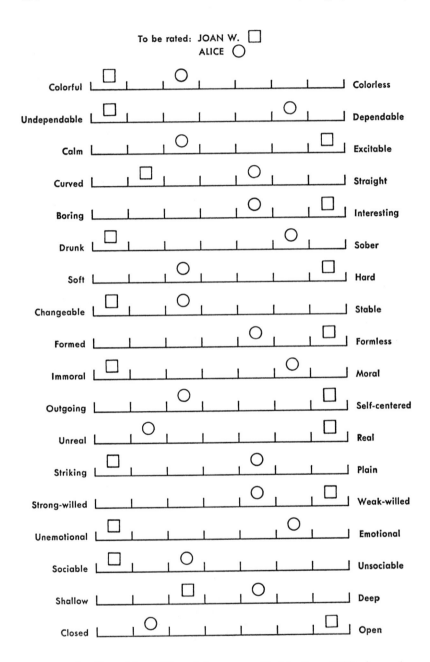

FIG. 10. Profiles of JOAN W. and ALICE provided by Joan Whitmier under hypnosis.

prived her of their mother's attention and love. She also affectionately recalled her grandfather as "the one I loved the most. He was just the loving kind. He always wanted me to sit on his lap and rock me. Mother never had time." When asked to examine her feelings toward her younger sister and to see if they had any application in the present, she immediately and for the first time confronted her hostile, jealous, competitive transference feelings toward her older daughter, Connie. The patient concluded the session with the recognition that a parallel existed between her relationship with Connie and her relationship as a child with her own mother: "This is the same reason I didn't obey my mother, because I felt that she didn't want me, so I didn't care if I did what she wanted or not, and that's the way with Connie. Connie felt like I didn't love her and so she didn't care whether she did what I asked her or not. But with her daddy, it was a little different. She felt like her daddy loved her more than her mother, and she would do the things he asked her."

A critical insight into her relationship with her parents occurred several weeks later. She was again reminiscing about her childhood when she recalled her fear of an older man, a friend of her father's, "who always carried a little snake in his pocket." Age regression was employed and almost immediately she re-experienced in detail a very traumatic incident at age four when this man had taken her into a barn and used her as a stimulant for masturbation. The patient reacted to recall of this experience with a sizable cathartic release.

The day following the above session, Alice, in a state of considerable agitation, requested another meeting. She stated that she was vaguely aware of another, related episode but that it had proven elusive to recall. Hypnosis allowed her to immediately recapture in convincing detail an experience from age five. She vividly recalled being fondled and then ejaculated upon by her alcoholic father. Alice went on to again connect this episode with her hatred of her husband, her hostility toward her mother for not having protected her, and the attraction felt for her lover — like her grandfather, he had loved her for herself, not sex. The next few sessions brought increasing expression of homicidal feelings toward her husband and an exploration of the following event which had precipated her hospitalization.

One night, when Alice and her husband were sleeping apart as usual, Connie came to her room crying and stated that she was afraid of her father. Instantly Alice *knew* that Frank had molested the girl and went into the living room to accuse him. At this moment, without any awareness of its source, she had remarked, "I know just how she feels because my father tried that on me once." Her husband vehemently denied the accusation but she remained adamant, felt physically ill, and was possessed of an intense hatred for him. "I told him I wanted to kill him. That a man who does that to his daughter isn't fit to live!" In the next couple of weeks an effort was made to work through this insight and while recall of the childhood experience raised doubt in Alice's mind regarding the validity of her interpretation, she remained highly ambivalent.

The last major therapeutic progress was made in the exploration of the meaning of her seizure pattern, and came about as the result of a pending visit of her ex-husband which precipitated the first seizure since she had begun hypnotherapy. Hypnosis was used to regress her to the time of each of a half-dozen seizures. The seizures were triggered off by direct suggestion and a detailed analysis was then made of the circumstances surrounding each event. The recurrent theme was a conflictual situation associated with overwhelming feelings of hopelessness and an appeal for help. The first seizure occurred two days after the situation in which Alice accused her husband of molesting their daughter. She had continued to press the issue and in a fit of rage he picked her up and threw her on the floor. "I remember thinking, 'Oh, my God, I can't move, my back's broken!' I couldn't move and I couldn't get up. *I couldn't get up*! And I crawled across the floor, got to the phone, and called the police. And he just stood there and looked at me!"

Additional questioning in a later session also elicited the fact that an older sister had always been subject to "spells" and even as a young girl Alice had the assignment of sitting on this sister's feet until the tremors passed. Alice's seizures thus became her means of escaping from an impossibly desperate situation.

Unfortunately, this promising therapeutic beginning did not result in lasting improvement. Despite everything, the patient had never relinquished her wish for a reconciliation with her ex-husband; it was truly a situation in which she couldn't live with or without him. She prevailed upon the therapists to effect a meeting with him for the purpose of exploring this possibility. While expressing a desire to cooperate, Mr. M. voiced his complete exasperation and refused even to consider the eventuality. Alice interpreted this action as one more in a long line of rejections and reacted accordingly. She became dispirited and depressed, lost her motivation for therapy, and her mood fluctuated widely and rapidly. She now openly expressed hatred of hospitalization and at the same time was exceedingly fearful of the prospect of discharge. She associated increasingly with another female patient, Maxine, whose behavior and dynamics were somewhat similar, and with her discussed the possibility of suicide. Alice also resumed the affair with her former lover. One weekend she went home with Maxine and the two of them actually made a half-hearted suicidal gesture.

The final episode occurred about one month later. Maxine signed herself out of the hospital "against medical advice" and sought electroshock from a private psychiatrist. After a series of six EST she returned to the hospital for a triumphal visit in a highly euphoric state, which she represented to the other patients as miraculously reinstated, radiant mental health. Alice thereupon demanded a similar treatment, and after some hesitation it was decided to administer a course of hypnoshock (Schafer, 1960; Guido and Jones, 1961). One actual full convulsive shock was administered, and thereafter a series of seven simulated shocks were instituted through hypnotic regression back to the original experience. After the first three "shocks" Alice felt well enough to go on an extended leave to her parents' home; the remainder were administered on an outpatient maintenance basis over a period of two months. Apparently Alice experienced her first shock as different from the ones which followed (Fig. 11).

A six-month followup revealed that Alice had maintained her improvement at least to the extent of remaining out of the hospital. She had married her lover, but unfortunately she contaminated a modern "miracle cure" when she and her new husband went to a private sanitarium and received several electroshocks in an effort to resolve marital discord.

Alice gives every evidence of developmental arrest at a very early age. As with the classical hysteric, she is characterizable as naive and suggestible, unreflective and impulsive, and in her relationships she is childishly clinging, affect-laden, and unstable. There is a powerful capacity for dramatization, and aggressive impulses are repressed and displaced. A prominent feature of Alice's pathology is an intense and protracted autonomy-dependency conflict. She vacillates perpetually between a childlike dependency and a facade of responsible adulthood, wallowing in indecision and ambivalence. Alice's intense frustration of early dependency needs is reflected in her life's task of searching for another person who will assume responsibility for solving her problems. The dependency and passivity expressed in this solution contributes to the fact that the hysteric is typically female and the problem-solver a male. Her marriage at age 14 was an early manifestation of this form of problem-solving.

Table 11 depicts the differences in the meaning of 12 concepts rated on the semantic differential over the three and one-half months of psychotherapy. The most decided feature was a wholesale flooding of hostility toward the husband ($D = 16.22$) and to a lesser extent toward the father ($D = 9.90$). The differential rating of MOTHER remains more or less neutral, while the rating of the concept GRANDFATHER was extremely positive. Some question of reliability may be raised. The ACTUAL SELF concept,

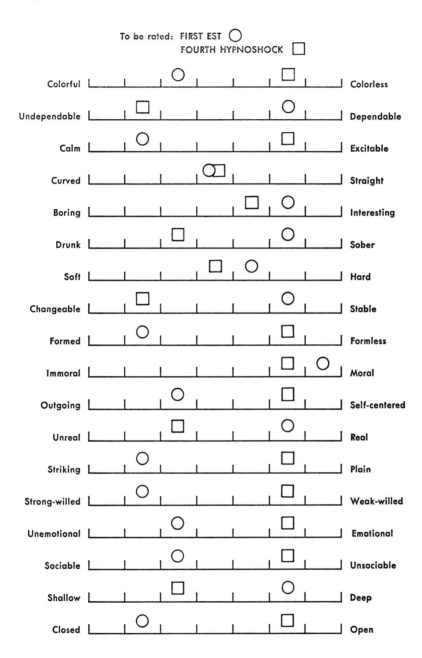

FIG. 11. FIRST EST (April 15) vs. FOURTH HYPNOSHOCK (April 22) on the semantic differential (D = 10.82).

TABLE 11. Differences in meaning of 12 concepts over four months of psychotherapy.

Concept	Difference in Rating
MEN	6.08
MOTHER	4.90
WOMEN	8.78
CONNIE	5.66
YOUNGER THREE GIRLS	4.35
FATHER	9.90
MAXINE	6.58
HUSBAND	16.22
THERAPIST	5.00
GRANDFATHER	4.24
ACTUAL SELF	5.66
IDEAL SELF	4.00

rated only three days apart (March 2 and again on March 5), reveals a marked degree of discrepancy, which casts some doubt on the consistency of all the measures; however, this item seems to reflect the tenuous self-concept of Alice, vacillating almost moment to moment (Fig. 12).

Alice seems attracted to men as a source of security rather than for sexual satisfaction; that is, she searches for the "good father," a tender, impotent male who, like grandfather, will comfort, caress, and provide for her without the burden of sexuality. Hers is a pseudosexuality in the sense that sex is viewed as a necessary evil, the price exacted from the female for need satisfaction from the male. In highly narcissistic fashion, Alice searches constantly for unqualified love but with an underlying conviction of eventual abandonment which contributes to her inability to reciprocate ("being loved is more important than loving").

Aggressive sexual advances, particularly from her husband, seem to have been unconsciously equated with the molestations experienced in childhood. It is a reflection of the strength of her dependency needs that Alice was willing to suffer 18 years of stressful married life and that only the direct reactivation of the oedipal conflict by her husband's assumed sexual advances to the daughter finally forced separation (and still Alice clung to the

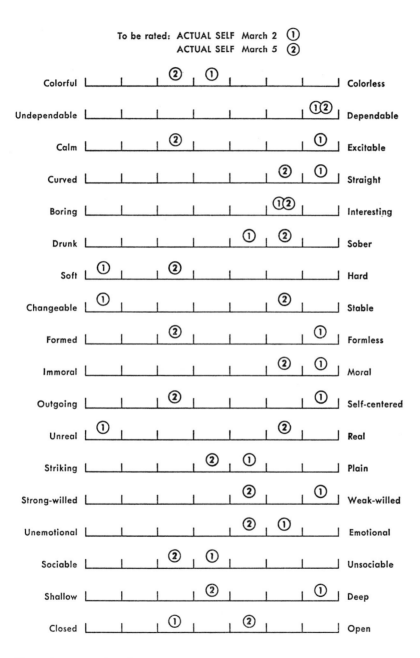

FIG. 12. Semantic differential ratings of ACTUAL SELF obtained three days apart ($D = 11.26$).

possibility of reconciliation). It is also noteworthy that despite the marked resentment felt toward her husband, the thought of sharing him precipitated an intense sibling rivalry with her own daughter.

Alice appears to have learned a generalized reliance on the repressive defense mechanism early in life as a way of grossly narrowing and constricting a threatening world into a more manageable form. The white dog dream graphically represents her effort as a young girl to distort and repress (shut the door on) unpleasant reality. Now, years later, Alice continues in her attempt to reject threatening reality but succeeds largely in disrupting her ability to "feel like a real person." Both of the patient's major symptoms, her seizures and the associated feelings of unreality, are comprehensible in terms of her excessive reliance upon this mechanism.

It seems a reasonable assumption that people strive toward coordinated, integrated, and consistent behavior. Experience can be handled in three ways: it is consciously symbolized and made meaningful, it is ignored and unrelated to the self-system, or it is disowned and distorted. Maladjustment ensues as a consequence of a basic incongruence between experience and the self-structure. In Alice's case, an independent existence entails responsibility and responsibility stimulates anxiety; however, to avoid responsibility as a wife and mother, particularly in view of the extreme condemnation of her own mother, causes severe guilt. Because her answer is to engage in efforts at wholesale repression, there is no role in which she can be a genuine person. Current efforts at dissociation are flamboyantly represented in the depersonalized personality fragment of Joan. In this embryonic double personality, Joan is the typical *black* (little girl) vs. *white* (Alice) which Osgood and Luria dealt with in the "Three Faces of Eve" (which were really just two aspects of the same personality).

Alice's seizures represent a prostration in the face of danger which annihilates the threatening perceptual image by temporarily rejecting consciousness itself, a mechanism not too dissimilar to the device of slamming an imaginary door in a dream. As with most symptoms, her seizures doubtlessly have multiple determinants; they certainly represent an expression of complete impotence and an appeal for help in a motoric manner; they are an expression of aggression in the form of an accusation ("Feel guilty, look what you have done to me!"); and finally, they seem to be a pantomimic repetition of traumatic physical and sexual assaults, possibly in an attempt at mastery.

It might be re-emphasized in closing that the favorable prognosis of the hysteric is largely illusionary. Freud acknowledged in the *Studies in Hysteria* (Breuer and Freud, 1950) that psychotherapy can sometimes effect dramatic changes in the symptom picture, but the underlying character structure remains largely resistant to radical alteration. Psychotherapy, of course, is a highly reflective exercise requiring that a patient assume increasing responsibility for his own thoughts and actions, but experientially speaking, the hysteric has forsaken the world of reflection for impulsive action. Personal responsibility is discounted so that things "just happen," seemingly at the instigation of others or impersonal events. Resistance to psychotherapy was therefore to be anticipated, and in this case, the patient's preference for hypnotherapy by a male therapist is recognizable as an obvious expression of her ever-present desire for a magical cure by the fear-provoking, omnipotent male. It may be further conjectured that Alice's willingness to relinquish her repressive controls initially were not entirely a healthy effort at integration, but were also an expression of her willingness to again "pay the price" in terms of the coin demanded in order to attain satisfaction of her gross dependency needs.

III. JOSÉ

The patient was a Mexican-American, aged 26, employed as a hospital recreation worker. Two interviews were spent in a conventional (nonhypnotic) attempt to explore the patient's precipitating complaint of "stuttering." Reluctantly but nevertheless persistently, she alluded to her unhappy marriage. Following is a verbatim account of the third session in which the attempt was made to focus on the problem that actually brought her into therapy.

P: I've been thinking about our talk yesterday, and about this "not listening habit" or whatever you call it. I wasn't aware of it. Sometimes I hear the words and I shut them out of my mind. I either misinterpret them or something. Or some part of me starts to answer without taking account of the words. So I tried to think about when I did this the most and I remember that I did it in connection with men, with boys back in school. I dated about 20 guys the first year in college, and I didn't get involved with any of them and in looking back, I realize that some of them tried to say something to me, but I did not listen. I either joked or I tried to put it in the right way. So the next question is how did Doug get through to me? Why didn't I listen to the other men, because they were a threat to me some way? And why wasn't Doug a threat to me? And the answer would be that he isn't a man, that he is a boy and as a boy he didn't threaten me? And why would I feel that men are a threat to me?

T: Well, it seems to me that you have taken some pretty large steps here. That is, you started off with why you seemed to be selective of what you listened to, and you've come up with a fairly profound analysis of it. I wonder if you can share with me how you arrived at these conclusions.

P: Well, it's very funny. My son played with some of my class books yesterday. When I came home, they were on the table and as I started to put them away, I looked through them and tried to pick out which of the men I had gone with in school. And then I thought why had I chosen Doug out of all the others who had a good future, some dentists, teachers, etc. So I wondered why did I choose Doug over all of them. And then I remembered, each time one of the men or boys or whatever you want to call them, tried to tell me that he could go for me, or get serious with me, I just joked! I remember other instances when they tried to get serious with me, and I just didn't care, I just didn't listen.

T: They wanted to be serious in their relationship with you, but you wouldn't allow it?

P: No. I was proud of the fact that I did not let them hold hands with me or kiss me, and I was keeping myself pure for my husband. But now I see that I was afraid of them, I didn't feel any emotion for them at the time.

T: Is the basic question here that you are asking yourself why you picked Doug when there were other opportunities which now in retrospect might have been better for you?

P: Well, it started in wondering why I shut myself out from other people sometimes, in what instances do I do it, and then it came down to Doug. Well, why didn't I shut myself from Doug?

T: There must have been something special about him that allowed him to get through to you.

P: I thought about that and it is either one of two things: either he is not a threat to me or he was very insistent. When Doug wants something, he will insist and insist and insist and just get it. But even so, if he was a real threat to me, he would not be able to get through to me, I don't think. So I don't know, it could be that he was so insistent, or that he was not a threat to me. And another interesting sideline to this is that I always thought that I wanted to marry a man who was most like my father. Doug is just as far away from my father as any man could be.

T: Did you actually end up with a person who was completely different from what you thought you wanted to marry?

P: Yes, that I wanted to marry. And that type can't be the kind who would scare me or threaten me.

T: What do you think the nature of the threat is that you're referring to here.

P: Well, one of the answers is that emotionally I am at a tomboy stage. I never had a chance to go through a tomboy stage; I was reared in a Spanish home. The men and the girls don't mix. So that could be one of the reasons. Or that I want unconsciously to be a man, and the men, they would threaten me. Yet I enjoy being with them, I enjoy their company much more than the company of girls. But when I saw that they wanted to get serious, then I shied away. As friends, fine, but not anything serious. And that would go along with my shying away from any physical contact with them, like holding hands, kissing, so forth and so on. But I don't see, I am a woman! I enjoy sex life. If I wanted to be a man, I wouldn't enjoy sex life, I don't think, I would be frigid, maybe.

T: Maybe. I don't think that you can necessarily say that.

P: If I wanted to be a man, I would take, what's the opposite of passive? [T gives the word "aggressive"] yes, I would be aggressive in the sex act, and I am not, I am passive and I enjoy it.

T: You want the man to make love to you?

P: That's right. I take part in it, but more in the passive way, at least in the start. Passive, in that I don't make the first move.

T: How do you feel now at this moment? You don't feel particularly anxious at the moment or under any sort of pressure?

P: No, not right now. At first when I discovered this blind spot or word blocking, I was very anxious, and I wondered how could I have done it? But my thoughts turned to now, how can I become a more mature person emotionally, if that's my problem.

T: You're still not certain as to what your problem is? You see, it strikes me again that you came in a couple of sessions ago, saying that you had this speech difficulty, and wanted to do something about that. And then you said that you felt resentful that we delved into this relationship with Doug. Yet I think it's also quite apparent that I don't push you into talking about these things — you do it spontaneously. I asked you, "Why do you think that you're selective in what you hear?" And you go home, you think about it, and then you again proceed to talk about your relationship with Doug, why you selected Doug, and why you didn't choose other men, what this meant to you. You see, you're the one who goes off talking about something other than this verbal blocking.

P: It all started because I wanted to know why I was resentful, why I did *not* want to talk about it.

T: So you can say that you came in and said initially that your problem was that of wanting to speak plainly. Either you're avoiding talking about your speech problem or this is somehow all related to it.

P: It must be related to it. It must be because it isn't that I don't want to talk about my stuttering. I do, but somehow or other, this seems to be the background for it. I can't think of anything else that would relate to my stuttering.

T: I'm not saying that this is necessarily bad that you're delving into this other material. All I'm asking is that you face up to the question as to what is the problem. What is the problem that you really want to work on?

P: The stuttering! Or when you put it that way, no. See, I answered it again without really giving it thought. The stuttering is a superficial problem. The other is an emotional problem which goes much deeper than the stuttering. Right? On the other hand, one could be a symptom of the other.

T: Well, which is the symptom of which? Do you think if your speech were improved that this would improve your relationships with Doug and men in general, or do you think if your relationship with Doug were improved and your relationships with men, that your speech might improve?

P: Well, I would say "no" to the first one, and "no" to the second one. I want to say "no" to the second one, but that doesn't make much sense because it has to be either one or the other.

T: Can you think of an alternative?

P: No.

T: Well, unless there is no relationship between the speech difficulty that you feel that you have and the security of your relationship with your husband. If there is no relationship, then you could say "no" to both.

P: All I know is that I expected to stop stuttering when I got married, when I got the emotional security that I wanted, and I think that I stuttered less when I was going with Doug when his affections were obvious.

T: Well, you mentioned that before. When you were going with Doug, you didn't stutter as much, and as you say, you expected when you got married and felt secure this difficulty would disappear.

P: Felt *more* secure. He was giving me deep emotional security at the time.

T: Well, then, let's go back again to your selection of Doug. Can you sit back and relax and just try to associate as to what Doug was to you, what he meant to you, why you preferred him?

P: It's very funny. I can tell just exactly what attracted me to Doug. We were going swimming, and I was with some other fellow and he was with a blind date. And we had our bathing suits under our clothes, and when he took his clothes off, I remarked what a nice body he had, and that's the first thing that I liked about him. At first, when we were first going together, I knew that we could never be married, because his background was so different from mine, there was no possible way, but then as we went together more and more, I didn't think of the differences. But there is a very great physical attraction at first, and maybe it's still there. Above everything else, and maybe that's all there is there, the physical attraction.

T: You still find sex as satisfying with him?

P: Yes, very much so. And then, of course, if that is what attracted me to him, I was a very immature person emotionally, and still am.

T: Do you worry a great deal that you're not as mature as you might be?

P: I used to think that I was mature, it's just since yesterday that I have given it thought, and I have come to the conclusion that I am very immature, that I must be operating at the level of a 14- or 15-year-old. So that's why I was attracted to him because we were at the same level emotionally.

T: So that he is in contrast to these men that you might have married, as you put it earlier?

P: Yes, he is in contrast to them. There's another thing, too, that helps me to come to this conclusion. When I talk about men, I hesitate to use the word "men," I would like to say "boys," but I am too old to talk about boys, they are not boys, they are men, yet I don't like to say men. It's as if the term "men" were a threat to me. I say men, I think men, I think of a big burly thing, while boys, they are not threatening.

T: You think there is a physical difference?

P: Between men and boys? I think it is deeper than the physical difference, the attitude, the expectations, the demands.

T: Well, tell me about your feelings of men and boys, the expectations, their attitudes and demands.

P: That's something else. Because I was brought up in a Spanish home, I had no contact with men at all. When I came to this country, this was the first time I had ever been away from my home, the first time I had ever done anything by myself, I used to think that men were different from girls. They thought differently, they felt differently, they acted differently, and it was a surprise to me to find that they were just like I was.

T: You attribute this to your Spanish background?

P: Well, I haven't given that any thought, but I had very little contact with the opposite sex and especially when we had moved from my home environment to Cuba. The first boy that I ever went with, we just wrote notes to each other, he was a student at the same school where my father was a teacher. My father said that if I did not stop going with him, he would have to quit his job, because it wasn't dignified for me to be going with a boy going to the same school where he was a teacher. I just didn't have a choice. And I was about 16 or 17 years old then. He was the first boy, I didn't care for him, but everybody else had a boyfriend so I wanted him, too.

T: So you feel that you grew up in a deprived home, deprived in that you had no contact with males, and that somehow this had something to do with the threat that men pose to you, and your preference to relate to boys? What do you think of a man as doing to you? What are the threats that you are talking about?

P: I don't know that it is something he might do to me, or something that I may do.

T: Tell me about that.

P: That I may not behave myself if I were alone with a man. I always think well, why couldn't I go to a man's apartment? Why am I so scared at the thought of going to a man's apartment? It isn't what he might do, it's what I might do, so that *I* might give myself to him without his asking, even. So that by my actions, my words, I might imply that I want him to do that, and yet be afraid at the same time.

T: A man will threaten your control?

P: It isn't the thought of going wild, it is not behaving, of giggling and being afraid that he is going to become intimate with me; I don't know, my thoughts are not clear on that.

T: Well, let's talk about boys, then. What's the difference in being alone with a boy?

P: A boy is a child.

T: And a child is someone you can control, isn't he?

P: Yes, a child does something he shouldn't do, you can slap him on the hands, and also this person is more like me.

T: What's the importance of this boy being like you?

P: The fact that subconsciously I want to be a man.

T: Where do you get this idea?

P: Well, not lately, not since I grew up. But when I was a child, I preferred playing with boys, I was very little, under seven or eight years old. And then I stopped because we moved. But I wanted to be a boy. Now I understand that a lot of girls go through that stage, that's called the tomboy stage; now it could be that I didn't have time to grow out of that because the war broke out, we moved out of our environment into another country, and I did not have a chance to continue in that stage and to get it out of my system. So I could be in that stage of still wanting to be a boy.

T: What does being a girl mean to you? What is a girl, what is a boy?

P: You mean a boy and a girl or a man and a woman?

T: Tell me about all four of them.

P: I know that being a boy at the time was the freedom that you had; also, I resented the fact that the girls had to wait to be asked, while the boy could go up and ask. He could choose, but the girl could not. She had to wait to be chosen. Sometimes during the sex act, I would wonder what the man would feel, I have tried to put myself, in my mind, in his place. What do you feel when you reach orgasm? When I reach orgasm, I enjoy it very much. A girl is a soft thing. She is weak, dependent, she looks up to the boys; the woman, she is stronger, but she is still weaker than the man, depends on him for support, advice, guidance, looks up to a man, it's very important that she look up to the man, because I looked up to my father, and yet the man I married, I do not look up to. And a man is a tower of strength, he is considerate, almost like a father. I see the woman as being the flighty one and the husband the steady one in the marriage. The boys are the rambunctious type, jumping, shouting, playing, getting his legs skinned, while the girl sits back with the doll and plays house. That's how I see the four of them.

T: There are a lot more limitations in being a girl than a boy?

P: Uh-huh.

T: And if you order them in terms of strength, then it's girl, boy, woman, and man?

P: Yes. And here's where the trouble can come, that in my marriage I have to be the strong one. I make the decisions, I pay the bills. Not that Doug can't do it, he does not want to do it. Even when we were separated, the moment that we came back together again, he sent me all the bills to pay. I pay all the bills, and then when there was a loan to be made, I used to go by myself, but now I have Doug go with me. I still do most of the talking, so in a way, I am the man of the house, I wear the pants. From birth, I've been trained to look up to the man and have him be the head of the house. So why didn't I choose a man that would do that? That's what it boils down to. What's in me that made me choose someone who was weak, emotionally immature, and far my inferior intellectually?

T: In other words, you now find yourself in a situation where, as you put it, you have to wear the pants in the family, you assume the responsibility, he leans on you, and you feel insecure in the situation. And that is the question, why did you put yourself in this situation?

P: My home was a strict one, and I was rebelling against my father. That's my pat answer. Is it the right one? Because he was as strict as any man can be.

T: How would you like to have married a man who was as strict as your father?

P: I wouldn't like it, I would rebel. I want some freedom of my own. No, I wouldn't like it. I have thought of that. I don't want a man to tell me what to do all the time and make all the decisions for me. No. I don't want that. I want freedom of my own. Yes, I want somebody to rely on, to depend on. I want to stand on my own feet; I want him to stand on his own feet. I have to be careful how I answer because so many times you say something and another part of me will answer without thinking. But I am thinking now.

T: Were you suggesting that perhaps Doug appealed to you for a number of reasons, one of which was that this was a boy who would not control you in the sense that your father had, that you could control him to a certain degree?

P: It seems that way. He controls me in a superficial way. For instance, if I want to wear shorts, and he says no, well that's it. Sometimes if it is important enough, I will argue about it and I will have my own way. But he does control me that way. But in general, intellectually, I am in control. I don't think I control him — "control," that has a lot of meaning.

T: I wonder if this is true, that he controls you to the extent that you work to please him, doing the things that you thought would please him so as to gain acceptance from him.

P: Yes.

T: And he controls you in a lot of other, minor ways, for example, this question of wearing shorts.

P: And not paying attention to other men.

T: But at the same time, when it comes down to the major responsibilities in the family, he relinquishes these to you and wants you to assume the responsibility there. Of course, in a sense, he is still controlling you there by *making you take these responsibilities.*

P: I hadn't thought of it that way.

T: Apparently this is something that is a threat to him, so he has you do it.

P: I hadn't thought of it that way either.

T: You see when a wife complains, for example, that her husband is weak, this immediately raises the question of whether she is keeping him weak.

P: I know what I have done to keep him weak, though. Before we were married, I had a job — he didn't. So we went up to Vermont where again I had my job, so I always made more money than he did. Then we waited for two years, and we came here. He was going to school, I was working. He was not studying, I was doing his homework, I was helping him with his classes. I was writing his themes, for a very stupid reason, because he wouldn't do it, that's all. I felt guilty that he had not finished school because when he was in school, we were not supposed to date because he was on a basketball scholarship; he did date me anyhow. He did not get his scholarship renewed, so I was bound and determined that I was not going to be superior to him in education. I was very anxious for him to finish school.

T: And so you did his school work for him?

P: Yes. Isn't that silly! Even now, in the mornings, he is very hard to get out of bed; what I ought to do, if he doesn't want to get out of bed is say, "O.K." No, I get mad and make him get out of bed. I treat him like a child.

T: Because as you said a few minutes ago, he is a boy, and yet you complain of feeling insecure because of the fact that he isn't a man.

P: Well, then, the next thing is that if I am unhappy in my marriage, it is my fault. It is my own shortcomings.

T: Except that you are thinking in terms of blaming someone.

P: Yes.

T: Well, does it make any sense for you to blame Doug?

P: I used to. In fact, up until yesterday. But now I see that it goes back to me, that I am the one. It is true that he is emotionally immature, but so am I. And one thing stands out, that he has made a much better adjustment than I have.

T: In what ways?

P: He is happy. If you were to talk to him for any length of time, he would strike you that he is happy, he is satisfied with what he has. He makes no other demands. He doesn't want any more out of life than what he has. But I am always striving for something more.

T: So being a striver, you said that you were bound and determined that he was going to finish his schooling, because you didn't want that much of a discrepancy between the two of you.

P: I didn't want him to feel inferior to me.

T: So you must have felt that he was inferior without this schooling.

P: Yeah. I know that I am smarter than he is. I was all the time an honor student. In college, he just barely got through, and he always

managed to flunk one or two courses every year. I knew that before we were married, too. Are we still talking about what I came
to talk about, or are we way out in left field?

T: Well, the question is, as we have been asking ourselves in all three
sessions, what is your problem? How can we answer it until we
know what your problem is? Why are you here talking?

P: Because I want to get rid of my stuttering.

T: O.K. Let's stop at that point now instead of pursuing what we have
been talking about. Your stuttering or blocking as I would call it
is a pretty big thing to you.

P: It is becoming less and less the more we talk. I can say in my soul,
deep down, that isn't so important. That it's the other that is the
main thing. My stuttering is a matter of vanity.

T: It's a pretty superficial thing in the balance of things.

P: Yes.

T: Do you think you've stuttered very much this hour?

P: Not too much. In some spots I did stutter. What did you think?

T: I don't see much difference in all three sessions.

P: Really?

T: Where do you think we ought to go from here, or do you think we
ought to go any place?

P: I still would like to try to be hypnotized.

T: Why?

P: Because to me it is such a simple way, like abra-cadabra, done!
We could go on and keep talking, but that would take a long time.
I suppose that would be good, but it's time which you don't have.

T: Well, don't put the responsibility on my shoulders. Let's say that
this would involve a lot of talking about things which might not be
too pleasant for you.

P: No, they would not be pleasant, I am sure, or would they? Would
I be glad to talk about it, get it out of my system? I would like to
face myself. It is true that I felt some reluctance coming when I
thought about the talk with you today.

T: You were reluctant to come?

P: I was reluctant at the thought of talking to you today. I wanted to
come and also I had a feeling that I did not want to talk about it
any more. I wanted to drop it. It's true that things that are unpleasant to me, I do not want to face them, or talk about them.

T: Going back to the reasons why you came in, I don't think there is
any simple answer, there are always two dozen reasons why people

come in. You don't just come in to therapy and say, "Well, I don't know why I'm here." So, you always pick out some reason.

P: Whether it's the real one or not?

T: Yes, certainly, but I understand perfectly well that this may not be *the* problem that you really want to talk about when you do come in, do you see? Because many people come in with a real problem and a surface problem. They began talking about the surface problem before they open up and talk about their real problem. Does that distress you?

P: It amazes me, how can you do this to yourself? It makes me mad!

T: Well, you're going to have about two weeks to think about this, since you're going away on vacation. So why don't you weigh it in your mind, think back over these sessions and try to make some decision about what your problem is and whether you do really want to work on it. Now, as far as your speech is concerned, I have something here which I would like to share with you. I recorded this session for you to listen to and I think it will convince you that you don't really have a speech problem.

At the conclusion of this session, the patient was asked to rate herself and other significant persons on the semantic differential (Table 12). The first thing to be noticed about the ratings is

TABLE 12.

Distance measures (D) of each of eight concepts with every other on the semantic differential.

	BROTHER	MYSELF	MOTHER	THERAPIST	DOUGLAS	FATHER	IDEAL	NEGATIVE
BROTHER	—							
MYSELF	11.83	—						
MOTHER	12.29	11.18	—					
THERAPIST	17.29	9.38	13.38	—				
DOUGLAS	17.97	13.08	10.72	9.75	—			
FATHER	17.18	10.20	13.27	5.92	8.72	—		
IDEAL	17.69	10.05	13.78	6.16	8.12	6.48	—	
NEGATIVE	15.07	17.92	14.42	20.81	19.67	20.49	20.40	—

again their absolute size reflecting the subject's use of the extreme units (1–7 and 2–6). THERAPIST and FATHER are somewhat similar and the husband, DOUGLAS, is surprisingly fairly identical. Using the IDEAL and NEGATIVE concepts as reference points, these first three concepts are much closer to the IDEAL than the

NEGATIVE self rating, while BROTHER and MOTHER have definitely more negative connotations, almost equally ambivalent; the MY-SELF concept is much more positive than either of these latter two, but less so than the original three.

In the fourth session, hypnosis was introduced into treatment. She was encouraged to relax, enter into hypnosis, and at this time she slipped spontaneously into a moderate-level trance and in this state demonstrated considerable aptitude for symbolic fantasies. The patient was stimulated to initiate a dreamlike, self-directed fantasy and to respond to it with a continuing projective self-structuring, so that she became progressively more immersed in an increasingly realistic fantasy experience.

She visualized that she was in a large "living room" furnished with "period pieces." There was a hallway leading from the living room but she found herself reluctant to enter it. When encouraged to do so she reported many doors ranging on either side and a patio with a fountain in the middle. After wandering through the house for a while alone, the therapist suggested himself into the situation with her. He told her he was going to take her to a room in which was housed the thing that she most feared and was most reluctant to face. She permitted herself to be "dragged" into a room. She reported that it was a dungeon and a number of emaciated, nude men were chained to the walls. She noted one man in particular, very thin, with a long beard.

The therapist then suggested to her that she take him to another room in the structure, "one which was not so disturbing to her." She proceeded to take him up a long winding staircase to the top of a turret and from there showed him a beautiful sunlit landscape. Just prior to arousal she told about a door that fascinated her but which she could not enter. The therapist suggested that he had the key but she emphatically rejected this idea.

Upon being asked to arouse herself she resisted the suggestion saying it was too pleasant where she was. During this time she had been given a pad of paper and a pencil and she roughly sketched on it. Upon awakening she identified her sketch as a lion with a cigar in its mouth and possessed of a breast (see Fig. 13). She seemed to have little understanding of what this represented and it was suggested that she think about the meaning of the fantasy and the drawing in the interim. An appointment was made for Tuesday, five days later. At the end of the session she was asked to rate her feelings about the LION WITH A CIGAR (Fig. 14).

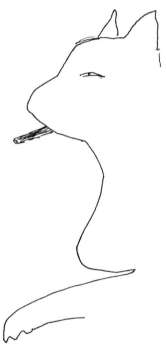

FIG. 13. Patient's drawing of lion with a cigar.

The next day, however, the subject called and urgently requested a session then rather than waiting until Tuesday. She reported that the night before she had gone to bed thinking about the session and had the following dream:

Doug and I were going somewhere in a car. We ran out of gas. We stopped at a roadside cafe. It didn't serve food or drinks. Somebody or something wasn't there and so we knew we would have to wait until Tuesday. Since we were out of gas we couldn't go on. I think we

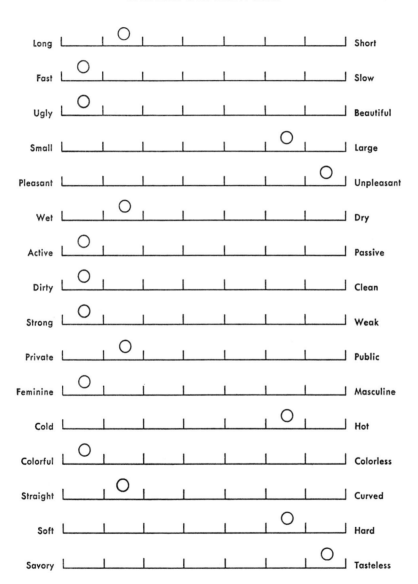

To be rated: LION WITH A CIGAR

FIG. 14. Semantic differential rating of LION WITH A CIGAR.

wanted to borrow some money. A colored woman ran the cafe. We wanted to go on but had to wait for the return of some guy to do so.

Upon awakening she recognized that her dream represented her impatience and desire to proceed with the therapy. She pondered the meaning of the dream fantasy of the previous day (as instructed) and came up with the following interpretation which seemed to occur spontaneously to her and which she had written down:

I called the structure a monastery. A monk is a castrated male; a monastery is a place for castrated males. Maybe the reason I did not want to leave [i.e., wake up] was because I was happy there. I took you to the tower with me to show you the wide view, maybe with the idea of making you stay there, that is, convincing you to stay in the monastery. The men in chains in the basement were not monks so they were not castrated, and perhaps that was why they were being punished. I felt no anguish on seeing them because I accepted the fact that they should be punished as the natural or normal thing. The man I had seen chained to the wall, fattened up and without beard, was undoubtedly Douglas.

It was interesting that it was only at your suggestion that you were with me at all. I became very disturbed when you offered a key to open the door because I knew that behind it was a statue of the Virgin Mary. Its silhouette reminded me of a big penis and I was horrified at the thought of your seeing it. It seemed a lack of property, ah, propriety.

For the first time she reported that in the courtyard the fountain had changed into a pit. When she looked in, an animal covered with horns had leaped at her. She now identified this creature as her father. "Another thing, the drawing of the lion chomping on a cigar became clear. It was to me the virgin engulfing, cutting off, and destroying the penis or the cigar. I really knew this during the last meeting but withheld it from you. I don't want to do the same thing next time." She was asked to draw the two conceptions of penis and the Virgin Mary (Fig. 15).

She then related that she had become increasingly aware of a "dark inner self." She spontaneously labeled it Josefa and then had thought, "That *really is* my name; that really is *me*." (It was a hated given name that she refused to accept.) It became apparent that Josefa represents her repressed feminine self in contrast to the masculine, assertive role that she has assumed. For example, she prefers being called José (a boy's name), wears her hair in a boyish bob, and thinks of herself as having a rather slight build and looking more like a boy than a girl. She spoke knowingly of José's fear of Josefa and the fact that Josefa would kill José if allowed dominance. It seemed evident to both discussants here that there is an intense inner conflict between the masculine and feminine aspects of this personality being represented in fantasy form.

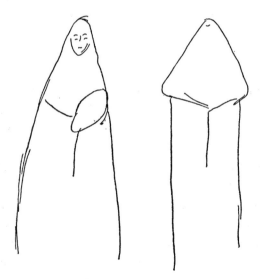

Fig. 15. The Virgin Mary and a penis.

José stated that following her writing down the foregoing interpretation, she had struck her hand into a fan. She immediately recognized that this represented a need for punishment and she had actually for a moment misperceived that three of her fingers had been cut off. She recognized that this action had been compulsively (unconsciously) determined. Finally, she reported a second dream but time did not permit examination:

A man had been in an accident and had burnt his hands badly. He wrapped something around my legs and when he took it off my legs had a black thick crust on them. He wanted to take it off with cotton but it hurt. He and I then went to a dance. He was naked and when he turned, it appeared he didn't have a penis, but rather looked like a woman — he had no hair in the pubic region. He had black spots on his body from the accident. The man was tall, strong built, blond, but his hand had been burnt off. He played the piano with artificial hands that looked like iron hooks. He played that piano with the lid closed over the keys and we all marvelled.

José was asked to awaken and to rate the following items on the semantic differential: VIRGIN MARY — GENERAL, VIRGIN MARY — FANTASY, PENIS, and VAGINA. She was unable to rate VAGINA and insisted on rating PENIS "as that belonging to a baby rather than a man." Only with insistence did she finally rate PENIS. At the end of the session she confessed that the items were rated according to Josefa's, not José's) disposition (Fig. 16).

The objective was to again capture the transformation of the latent content into a symbol, this time in the context of an actual clinical session, in contrast to the earlier experimental study of the hypnotic dream induction (e.g., NECKTIE into PENIS, pp. 22–24). The Virgin Mary as she is generally conceived (VIRGIN MARY — GENERAL) immediately undergoes a marked transformation in meaning when incorporated into the patient's fantasy (VMG:VMF, $D = 12.52$). When the rating of PENIS is compared to the two aspects of the concept, it is obviously much closer to VIRGIN MARY — FANTASY ($D = 8.66$) as contrasted with the ordinary meaning of the Virgin Mary ($D = 15.59$). It is also of interest that Josefa's original rating of PENIS "as that of an infant" (which the Virgin Mary holds in her arms) obtains a distance measure in relation to VIRGIN MARY — FANTASY of 15.43 vs. a distance of 6.93 in relation to VIRGIN MARY — GENERAL. Of course, a confounding fact was the patient's aware-

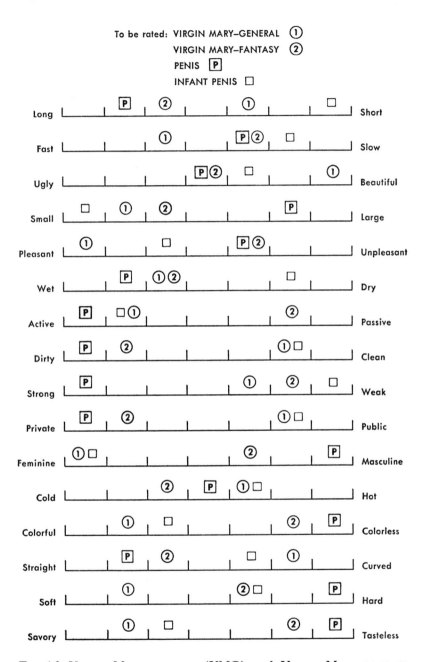

FIG. 16. VIRGIN MARY–GENERAL (VMG) and VIRGIN MARY–FANTASY (VMF) as contrasted with PENIS and INFANT PENIS.

ness of the identification of penis with the Virgin Mary in her fantasy, but again there is evidence of the symbol definitely moving in the direction of the underlying content.

On July 29, the subject reported three dreams that occurred on the weekend.

Diving to the bottom of a pool to retrieve something black some children had thrown in. Somebody was going to empty the pool, but I insisted on diving anyway. The pool was emptied afterwards. I was admired for my deed. [The last sentence had been scratched out by the subject on the paper on which she had listed the dreams.]

I was on one of the men's wards. One of my patients was showing me something, a new magazine or silver cup. We were alone in the dining room. The man wore black — he was a patient who sexually stimulated me. We were leaning against a table. He had his hand on my hip or side and it felt good. He didn't seem to notice how it affected me. One of the men on the ward was sitting on the floor against a wall, and he had a raw spot on a thigh, it looked like it had been burnt and had a dark edge around it. The attendant told me he had bitten himself.

There was a man in the room at the bottom of the steps. He was standing still, on the right, and he was laughing and leering at me. He was dressed in period clothes and there was something very white and bright about his face — his eyes, I think.

The patient began with the statement under hypnosis that the connection between the Virgin Mary and penis was a revelation. She questioned to whom the penis belonged. "Is it my recognition that I have no penis really?" She recalled her "fanatical Catholic training" in Mexico and her childish fear that God might reveal himself to her while she slept. She also recalled the slip she had made substituting "property" for "propriety." She questioned whose *property* the penis really was. She went on to contrast the fact that in her fantasy the penis had been located downstairs behind a locked door while the vagina was upstairs in the sunlight in peace. At the same time she recognized that the tower or penis intruded itself into the landscape and she recalled that she and the therapist did not stand near the window. "Am I afraid to get too close to the window, afraid of falling? The 'you' in my fantasies is not you [i.e., the therapist] but the masculine side of me. I took 'it' to the tower to show a wonderful view. The tower obviously represents a penis and the window a hole or the vagina so that I was saying to my masculine side, 'Let me have the freedom and happiness of being a woman,' while also asking him to stay in the monastery where he was a castrated male."

She then discussed part of her dream reported in the second hypnotic session. She questioned whether the tall, blond man was not her masculine self. She recalled she held him by her right hand. To her, right means masculine and left means feminine. In associating to it she came to the conclusion that music on a closed piano represented love, but an unnatural love expressing her concern over masturbation, frigidity, and unresponsiveness. The hands replaced by hooks suggested that they were not of the man's own flesh and blood and, as such, were a denial that she masturbated with her own hands. Rather, this was her masculine side making love to the feminine side.

Discussion then turned to the two different aspects of her personality. She characterized José as strong and self-sufficient. She admitted frequent indulgence in compensatory, conquering, hero-type fantasy in which she would be recognized for her great deeds. In one recent fantasy she and several members of the Psychology Service, including the therapist, had been kidnapped and were tied up in an attic. She escaped and in a very dramatic manner killed four or five men who were going to rape her. She then recalled the dream in which a man was hiding at the bottom of the stairs, laughing and leering at her. He seemed to say, "You did what I wanted you to do." She was concerned that he might attack her. She recognized that on the one hand she had a strong desire to be raped and, on the other, reacted with murderous impulses. Josefa would give herself to him but José prevents it. José has the attitude, "The man has not been born who can rape me." The question of identity was discussed. She denied that this man represented the therapist, saying that in this situation the therapist had no gender. "I think of you as a rubber ball, I mean a rubber wall, off of which my feelings bounce."

The subject again turned her attention to the earlier fantasy in which she saw her husband in the dungeon, weak and sagging against his chains. Her attitude was, "He deserves to be there because he isn't any more of a man. He rejected me when I was most feminine, that is, when I was pregnant. Is it possible that I am denying him his masculinity or virility?"

The patient began hypnotic session IV by reporting a dream, but maintained it had no meaning for her. Asked to relax, she spontaneously drifted off into a state which she described as "extremely pleasant — like when I am in bed at night with Doug and he cuddles me in his arms. I feel so happy, complete, protected, confident — a feeling of being loved and wanted." Through suggestion, her sensations and feelings associated with this room were intensified. Her description suggested that it might symbolically represent the womb in which she felt completely secure. The therapist deliberately commented: "You make it sound *heavenly*." The patient responded immediately with a vision of the Virgin Mary, babe in arms, hand raised in a blessing. Suddenly it dissolved and was replaced by a penis. She had a strong negative reaction. "It's dirty, I don't want to see it, it's so big, it makes me feel so small, it takes up all of the room, it's big, filthy, dirty, lewd — the Virgin Mary hides it."

The suggestion was given that she regress in memory to the first time she ever thought and felt about the penis in this manner. She responded with apparent memory of watching her father wash himself in the bathroom. She described her thoughts as: "What is that? It's so big; it looks so black and dirty. It looks like a bowel movement." The father teased her, saying that it was something to eat, and laughed at her. The suggestion was made that she regress to the memory of the first time she became aware of the use of this organ. She responded with a memory of standing in her parents' bedroom when she was about three or four years of age. She was shocked at witnessing her father having intercourse with her mother. The father was seen on his knees over the mother who was lying on her stomach. As she watched the scene, the father's face became that of a wolf. She questioned anxiously, "How can Mother be so relaxed and happy when she has an animal on her back? She doesn't know he is going to eat her, sink his teeth into her neck, and snap her head off."

At this point she expressed herself as happy at the fact that the father was going to destroy the mother. "I don't like her. She is jealous of me. I want her to go away and then I'd have my father to myself. I'd take good care of him and make him happy. I could cook and we could talk and joke." Asked whether she could take care of him in all ways, the patient responded in a highly distressed tone, "No, no, no, not in bed!" This was followed by the seeming recognition that she could not really replace her mother. "I'd just be able to do the surface things. She'd do the complete *setting*."

The discussion then evolved around her relationship with Doug. She commented that she saw Doug as a little boy, perhaps about seven years of age. She had a fantasy in which she held his head to her breast and rocked and soothed him. But he rejected her, didn't want to be soothed. "He's just a little too old for me to rock him, he thinks it's sissy, he wants to go play with his friends. I want to love him, hold his head against my breast." The question was introduced regarding the contrast of breast love and genital love. Still in the mood of the fantasy she reported that she was "closed" to him. "A little boy can't play with his mother's vagina. If he tries, I swat his hand."

In hypnotic session V, the patient began with the statement that she felt an intense hatred for the therapist. She recognized that this hatred was irrational and that the therapist had done nothing to earn it and then recognized that actually she hated her husband, but there was danger in hating him so she displaced it onto the therapist.

In the prior session (IV) the patient had reported a dream, the essence of which was that she had lent some clothing to another girl, had received two items back, but the girl still had her red skirt. In company with another girl she went to the first girl's room in order to get the skirt. She found the room in a state of general dishevelment. While there, her companion sat on the bed while she browsed around the room. Finally she picked up a bottle and threw it through a mirror in a fit of anger. This act calmed her. During this action her companion watched her with a rather sad expression.

She stated that she had developed a number of insights concerning the dream. As usual, these developed spontaneously rather than as a result of any logical process. She recalled that in the dream she had felt very angry at the girl who had borrowed her skirt and not returned it. She remembered thinking, "She can't get away with it. Who does she think she is? She can't take my clothes like that." She also recalled that the room was in a mess with clothes piled high. Everything was in chaos. She found the skirt finally in a pile of clothing. Her companion was sympathetic but silent. She now recognized this girl as a twin sister, that is, "the other me — Josefa." She stated that there was some significance to the fact that the two articles of clothing that had been returned were a white sleeveless sweater and a black skirt. The only colored object in the dream was her skirt. She assumed that this matter of color in the dream had some significance but was unable to comprehend its meaning. She recalled stomping about the room and roughly searching through things and sweeping articles from the top of the dresser. Inside she became angrier and angrier. Finally she broke a mirror by throwing a bottle through it, leaving a gaping hole. She recalled that the bottle was shaving lotion. The action greatly reduced her anger.

She associated to the act of breaking the mirror and quickly came to the conclusion that the bottle was a symbol for the penis. She stated that the act of breaking the mirror represented an assault of rape. She questioned, "Do I have a desire to be a man; to push a penis into a vagina? Do I have a desire to commit rape, to hurt a woman, to punish her by disregarding her feelings? I have a feeling I would like to rip and tear and give vent to my anger like an animal that has been repressed."

These associations made her think again of the skirt. The skirt then developed a sexual meaning for her and as she pictured it, it turned into the head of a wolf with an open mouth which she then recognized as the vulva: "Like looking into the vagina. I am reflected in the mirror and by this action I am broken too, that is, broken by the bottle. Then only the other girl remains — the quiet, patient one — while the angry, loud one is destroyed. Somehow one of me has been destroyed by breaking the mirror. The girl in the mirror was ugly. Her face was contorted with rage. She looked more like an animal with her lips drawn and her teeth prominent — like a wolf." She was asked to sketch the scene under hypnosis (Fig. 17).

She then commented that the bottle of shaving lotion was similar to that used by her husband. This led her into a discussion of her feelings of revulsion when her husband occasionally asked her to engage in fellatio. She allowed herself to be persuaded to engage in the act but felt that it was of great indignity, that somehow it was degrading. The next association she had was the memory, recalled in the previous session, of watching her father

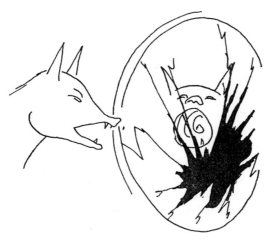

Fig. 17. Wolf in the mirror.

wash his genitals. She seemed to recall that she was impressed that it was dark in color. She asked her father what it was. He said it was something to eat. She seemed to feel that it looked or reminded her of feces. It was interesting at this juncture that several times in attempting to describe her feelings, she made another slip: "It's chocolate-covered, I mean colored."

The next association she had was another memory recalled in the previous session of seeing her parents having intercourse in which her father had mounted the mother from the rear. It then seemed as if these associations went into a meaningful pattern, namely, that in her little girl mind the penis was associated with feces, both by its color and shape and by the possible misconception that intercourse took place in the mother's anus. Thus, it became clear to the patient why the penis of her husband, which she acquainted with the dirty penis of her father, was so repulsive to her. This discussion then returned to the drawing she had once made of a lion with a cigar in its mouth. She then recognized this as being symbolic of much that had been discussed during the hour. The cigar represented a penis, but a black penis, depicting her confusion as to the nature of this object.

She turned her attention finally to identification of the three women in her dream. The first girl, Josefa, was characterized as

quiet, dignified, and feminine, a person who is calm and accepting because of her inability to do anything about the situation. The second was coarse, had prominent teeth, was loud talking, angry, and broad-shouldered — the masculine type. She is the animal one who destroys herself in the mirror. I wonder who the bottle was intended for. After the mirror is broken her reflection is destroyed, but the quiet one is still visible. The third girl [i.e., the absent borrower] is very attractive, has a nice figure, beautiful breasts. Now I am getting all confused. I can't understand the red skirt either. I wonder — is it like a red herring in order to draw attention away from something? When I think about it I get a very distasteful picture and that is of a used sanitary pad. I don't know what that could mean. The room is disarranged — the odds and ends, the things that don't seem to belong, I wonder if they don't represent my cluttered mind.

The subject was asked to rate the concepts of JOSÉ and JOSEFA on the semantic differential (Fig. 18). Once again, the ratings reveal the same dichotomy between the basic *white* (Josefa) and *black* (José) components. In the triple personality case of Osgood and Luria (1954), "black" was also quite masculine. In contrast to the original rating of MYSELF, the semantic distance to José is 7.65 and 13.82 to Josefa.

This was the fifth hypnotic and final session. She stopped coming to the interviews and she and her husband moved out of town shortly thereafter. In June of the following year, almost 11 months later, she paid the therapist a return visit. Her first statement was about how much he had helped her. She cited, for example, that "Now I just don't masturbate anymore — I just don't have the urge." This she related to the fact that José was no longer the ascendant personality, that she felt much more comfortable as Josefa now. "I also am no longer resentful when Doug doesn't show me any affection." She announced that they were separated and planned a divorce. At the same time it was apparent that she did not want to leave him, while she insisted that she would not go back unless he agreed to see a psychiatrist. The only answer she could give as to why she was so strongly attracted to him was "sexual satisfaction." In the next breath she confessed that she had entered into an affair with the husband of her best friend. This surprised her since it dispelled the illusion that her moral standards would always prevent her having such a relationship.

Discussion

In the attempt to reconstruct the background of the patient's problem, it was very clear that she was brought up in a strict Spanish-Catholic home with little opportunity for the usual heterosexual relations. What she knew about sex was learned largely from the chance observations of her parents, mixed with a great deal of vivid fantasy. The result was that she was confused about her own sexual identification. There were many hints of this in

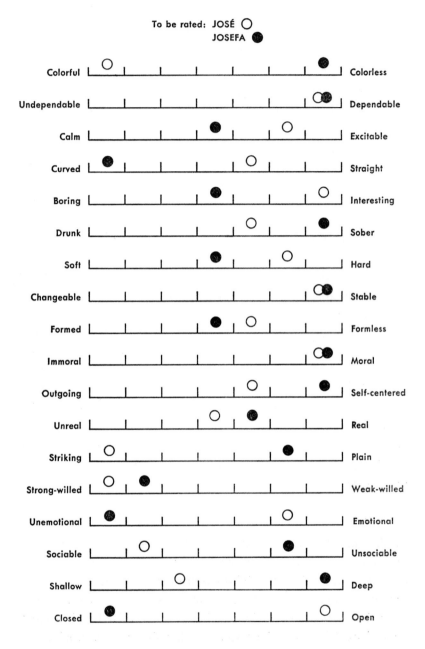

FIG. 18. JOSÉ:JOSEFA (D = 14.36).

the original discussions with her: she placed herself at the tomboy stage; she complained that a girl is faced with many limitations and said frankly that she preferred to be a man; she was attracted by the physique of her husband-to-be, but he turned out to be only a boy in the larger sense; in contrast, she knowingly rebelled against her authoritarian father and yet she did not like the responsibility that she had to assume in her married life, etc. Thus many of the ingredients of her problem were apparent by the end of the third session. The fact that she came back after a two-week vacation and again demanded hypnosis prompted utilization of this technique. Once hypnosis was induced she played out her problem in her dreams and fantasies to what was, for her, a satisfactory conclusion. She apparently knew all along that she would soon be leaving and hypnosis accelerated the process for her.

The dreams and fantasies of the patient immediately cast the conflict into a highly personalized meaning system for her. In her initial fantasy she described her wishful escape into religion. She pictured a monastery and the fact that she felt happy there as a woman, being removed from her sexual conflict. She described her husband as a noncastrated male who was confined in a dungeon, thus removing the threat of his sexuality, while the therapist who had originally optioned to place himself in the fantasy was recast by the patient as her masculine self to whom she pleaded for the right to be a woman. At the same time, she recognized the urgency of the conflict between the masculine and feminine parts of her personality. In real life she had assumed some of the trappings of the male. The question was, at that point, does the penis really belong to her? She was horrified at the sacred image of the Virgin Mary (her idealized feminine self) in the fantasy as being replaced by an ugly, lewd penis (the masculine self). At the same time she visualized a fountain or pit in the patio of the monastery, from which a monstrous creature leaped at her. She was puzzled by the eventual identification of the creature as her father. Following the hypnotic fantasy she drew a lion with a cigar, which she interpreted as a female lion devouring the penis. Finally, in making waking ratings on the semantic differential of the lion, she confessed that they were made by a "dark, inner self," Josefa, the female part of her nature. She felt extremely threatened, in that Josefa would kill her, José, if allowed dominance.

Her second symbolic experience was of a nocturnal dream which depicted her concern with autoeroticism which, however, she continued to project onto a dual personality. One role in the dream was of a tall, strong man whose hands and penis were destroyed in an accident, and the other person was herself. He played the piano with iron hooks and everyone was very impressed, especially because the lid was closed on the keys. The patient interpreted this as her masculine self making "unnatural love" (masturbation) to the feminine self. At the same time, she recognized that while Josefa had a strong desire to be raped, the masculine self, José, attempted to repress these impulses. Obviously, the patient's compartmentalization of the masculine-feminine aspects of her personality was most tenuous.

The third and last experience was of a second dream in which the patient had lent some feminine clothing to another girl and when it was not returned, both José and Josefa went to the girl's apartment. The patient recalled her confusion over seeing the father's genitals when she was a very small girl and of watching her mother and father engage in intercourse from the rear. These associations apparently were related to her sexual confusion in later years and were the basis of the symbolism depicting her father as a horrible creature in the fantasy. In relation to the dream, she said that José was increasingly angry at not being able to find the missing "red skirt" (which had a definite effeminate connotation) and finally, in a fit of rage, José picked up a bottle of shaving lotion and hurled it through a mirror. This the patient interpreted as an act of rape. Instantly José was destroyed by the action and "only the quiet, dignified, feminine person was left." At that juncture the patient left therapy. When she returned a year later, the patient confirmed that Josefa had maintained her ascendancy.

There are many questions left unaccounted for in this case and a more traditionally trained psychotherapist might well react to the fact that so many ends remain untied and so much is left unknown to him. Certainly the patient was far from being ideally well adjusted. Yet, this is a case where the patient utilized therapy to accomplish a primary objective and so far as one can believe her, she began to achieve her goal. In five hypnotic (eight total) sessions, she had begun to resolve her identification dilemma so that she felt able to function better and to make some additional progress on her own. If this surmise is true, then perhaps it is all that one can count on from a relatively intense, yet limited psychologic involvement.

The question is almost invariably raised: are such multiple or dual personalities artifacts of psychotherapy? Certainly the essence of the psychological treatment is to differentially reinforce certain aspects of behavior while minimizing others, a process which could conceivably enhance the differences which reside within all personalities. Presumably, hypnosis could encourage any dissociative tendencies, resulting in the gradual evocation of a fully developed secondary personality. Harriman (1943), for example, found that when he "erased" his subjects' primary personalities with hypnotic suggestion, they spontaneously developed secondary personalities to fill the vacuum.

On the other hand, it may be that dual personalities exist in much greater numbers than is generally supposed. Forty years ago, Alexander wrote:

Therefore, when I describe the superego as a person, and neurotic conflict as a struggle between different persons, I mean it, and regard the descriptions as not just a figurative presentation. . . . Furthermore, in the study of the neuroses there is no lack of such visible manifestations as a divided personality. . . . In contrast to the emphasis laid on the varying roles of the analyst in the transference situation, little has been said about the varying role of the patient who may present to the analyst not one personality but many. The mechanism by which multiple personalities are established is as yet unknown. One may ask whether all acts of repression may not involve the creation of a larval form of a secondary personality (1929, p. 55).

REPRISE

It is inevitable that the discussion of the genuineness of any behavior elicited by hypnotic suggestion concerns itself ultimately with the nature of hypnosis per se. In a sense the usual "hypnotic dream" can be regarded as only one variation of the hypnotically induced hallucination, and all hypnotic manifestations are related to this phenomenon. As Orne (1962) has written, "The process of trance-induction can be viewed as a gradual increase of potentiality to experience suggested alternations of the environment as subjectively real phenomena." In other words, a subject volunteers with a readiness to allow his perceptions to be manipulated, and the hypnotic induction procedure is carefully calculated to reinforce this conviction and to exclude intrusive, contravening thoughts. In this manner, "hypnosis encourages the relaxation of reality testing functions in areas designated by the hypnotist, so that typically a subject manifests the peaceful coexistence of logically discrepant perceptions" (Orne, 1962). Subjective images and ideation become confused with external events, which grade gradually into hallucinations as the subjective belief in the reality of the false perception increases.

Certainly the parsimonious explanation of hypnotic phenomena is that for whatever reason the subject is highly motivated to cooperate with the hypnotist (i.e., he is hypersuggestible), and the possibility exists that a patient will produce and respond to symbols with an intention of conforming to what he perceives to be the therapist's biases, prejudices, and predilections. Conversely, a trained hypnotherapist is keenly aware of this possibility; sometimes he capitalizes on it, and most of the time he tries scrupulously to avoid giving cues that could direct the patient. At the same time, most hypnotherapists become rapidly aware that the patient's compliance with his suggestions are more apparent than real.

The majority of the symbolic productions produced in this book are not "hypnotic dreams" but are largely spontaneous fantasies and nocturnal dreams and they are not usually the result of either a general or specific suggestion made by the therapist. The process with these cases was just the opposite of what Orne writes about in his chapter. It is true that the therapist may structure a selective inattention to external events and a guided awareness of potentially perceivable inner stimuli in the patient, but very seldom does he suggest the nature of a dream and certainly not the interpretation of the various symbols employed. Just as the hypnotic hallucination can result from a belief in the reality of calculative false perceptions, as it is used here, the hypnosymbolic phenomenon tries to tap the underlying meaning of the patient's subjective reality.

These three cases were deliberately chosen to represent contrasting problems, strategies, tactics, and goals and they are also intended to demonstrate the limitations as well as the virtues of brief, crisis-oriented hypnotherapy. The first case, of a war neurosis, is somewhat similar to what might be attempted by a behavior modificationist, with a minimum effort at exploring the patient's cognitive or meaning structure and a maximum effort in attempting to desensitize the patient. The second case of Alice M. utilizes multiple hypnotic techniques, only a few of which might be classified as actually hypnosymbolic in nature, but it is instructive of the wide variety of hypnotic tactics employed even though it was not a successfully treated case. The last case, José, utilizes the patient's motivation to work through her problem and the role of therapist is almost entirely as participant-observer of the process. A special value is that it does provide the occasion to contrast conventional psychotherapy with the utilization of the hypnosymbolic technique by the same patient-doctor tandem. Obviously, the approach is not restricted to palliative suggestion.

At the same time it should be equally evident that it is not a panacea; it does require a certain amount of skill and even daring to use the hypnosymbolic technique.

The semantic differential ratings serve to illuminate the clinical proceedings and, in some instances, to act as an evaluation of a case. The clearest evaluation is in the treatment of the war neurosis, in which three sets of the same 15 concepts were evaluated over the course of treatment. In the case of Alice, 12 concepts were evaluated over the course of four months of treatment; however, there is some question as to the reliability of the ratings. From a clinician's point of view, her ratings are of interest in contrasting ALICE with her dual personality JOAN, and in the comparison of the real electroshock treatment that was experienced quite differently by the patient from the hypnoshocks which were subsequently received. With José it was possible to obtain only one set of ratings, since she left therapy rather unexpectedly; nevertheless, inferences can be made from the one set. Clinical information is also obtained from José's rating of various symbolic expressions, such as the LION, José's and Josefa's ratings of the VIRGIN MARY and the latent content, and the differences between JOSÉ and JOSEFA, the masculine and feminine aspects of the same personality. Ratings like these should support the many different ways that clinicians can make use of the semantic differential in searching for the unique significance or meaning of the individual behavior disorder.

NINE   "Black Rover,
                                Come Over!"

INTRODUCTION

A frequently encountered problem in clinical practice is the
treatment of irrational phobic fears. The nature, depth, and duration of therapy naturally varies with the individual patient and
depends on a number of interrelated factors, such as the type of
phobia, the dynamic importance of the symptom, and the relation of the phobia to the personality structure of the patient. This
is a report of the brief, successful treatment of a phobic reaction
in which the patient's repressive defenses were penetrated, leading to a simple, convincing demonstration of the childhood learning of the phobic response and its subsequent ramifications. A
symbolic fantasy procedure, tailored to the patient's unique personality dynamics, was then instituted in order to consolidate the
obtained insights and further desensitize the patient to the fear-
provoking stimuli.

Primary reliance was placed on several innovations in hypnotherapeutic technique, including the fact that psychotherapy
contacts per se take such an infinitesimally small portion of a patient's time (one or two hours for a few weeks) that every attempt is made through hypnotic suggestion to make this a real
experience for the 168 hours of the week. The effort was made to

capitalize on the fact that this patient was a very well-organized individual and her diary attests to the success in making treatment an exceedingly important, if transitory, part of her life. This information provided by the patient also testifies to the validity of the content dredged up by the hypnotic procedures.

Session I, January 23

The patient, aged 45, an art instructor in a nearby women's college, appeared punctually in company with her husband. She explained that she had brought him since she feared that under hypnosis she might say something that the therapist later would not tell her. She stated that she had suffered an extreme fear of dogs since early childhood. Recently she had seen a movie, *The Three Faces of Eve*, and this picture had stimulated her to seek professional help. A solution to the problem was particularly pressing at this time because she wanted to get her daughter, Judy, a dog as a birthday gift two weeks hence. It was agreed that there would be a maximum of six or seven sessions. The time limitation was introduced to optimally mobilize the patient's motivation for early recovery (she had already stipulated two weeks!) and to avoid the long-term relationship involving strong dependency which sometimes develops in the treatment of chronic phobic reactions. At this juncture the patient was requested to rate several concepts on a form of the semantic differential.

The remainder of the session was spent in training the patient to facilitate relaxation and experience general hypnotic phenomena. It was suggested that she was lying in the bottom of a flat-bottomed row boat on a spring day, floating gently down a slow-moving stream. After approximately 10 minutes, it was suggested that she picture herself at the head of a flight of 10 steps leading down, that she was to imagine walking down these steps, that with each step she would become more relaxed and drowsy, and that finally at the bottom she would go completely asleep. She was then given the posthypnotic suggestion that in the future, when the therapist tapped on the desk twice with a pencil, she would go rapidly and deeply asleep. She was instructed to be amnesic for this suggestion. It was suggested that hypnosis would be a happy experience for her, that she would find it relaxing and would recognize that in this manner she was helping herself with her problems. She was then awakened.

The patient exhibited a typical reaction of most subjects upon first being hypnotized, that is, an expression of surprise at having been "fully conscious" throughout the whole procedure. She also was not amnesic for the suggestion to go to sleep at the tap of the pencil. In this instance the suggestion of amnesia obviously conflicted with the patient's stronger need to remember (attested to by the presence of her husband). This is one of the many examples of the fact that the hypnotized patient remains an individual with full rights and privileges. Nevertheless, when the therapist tapped the pencil, she went almost immediately into hypnosis. At the end of the session she asked the following question:

P: When I am able to go deep enough to go back and find out what my fear of dogs is, can you make a stop along the way?
T: Certainly, if you wish.
P: I haven't thought about it for a long time. About 10 years ago in the delivery room something happened that I tried hard to remember but I couldn't quite. I have been curious what it was I wanted so desperately to remember. I wondered if in going back 40 years one could make a stop back 10 years.
T: [Humorously] That should be only about one-quarter as difficult.

Session II, January 27

The patient arrived promptly and alone. She volunteered that her husband had thought the previous session was interesting and he regretted that he could not come today because of a conference. She also remarked, "Incidentally, I kept remembering your tapping on the desk over and over again. Ordinarily I would not remember a minor incident like that unless there was a good reason for it." The therapist then induced hypnosis by tapping the desk. The patient settled back and after several more taps went deeply asleep. Suggestions were given reinforcing the hypnotic effect of the taps. It was suggested that when she was as deeply asleep as she was the previous time, she was to signal. The staircase scene was then reinstated. It was suggested that she proceed down to the twenty-fifth step, "going much deeper all the time." As she proceeded, the suggestion was changed so that she was no longer going down steps but was in a descending elevator going rapidly past whole floors. Further suggestions were given to the effect that in the future at the given signal she would go quickly and deeply asleep. It was again suggested that the patient be amnesic for these suggestions. The patient was then awakened.

T: You appear puzzled about something. Is it a little hazy?

P: It is something about tapping on the desk. [Her voice trails off and she continues to look preoccupied.]

T: It bothers you when you cannot remember something?

P: Yes, it does. It bothers me when I cannot remember things.

T: Can you trust me in this situation that it is not always necessary to immediately recall everything?

P: Yes, I think so.

T: Just relax and see what happens when I tap the desk. [Taps. The patient immediately nods, relaxes, and falls asleep. She is then given a reassuring suggestion.]

Hypnosis can be frightening for some people, especially in the beginning because it requires that you give up some control, in a sense. This can be disturbing for people who pride themselves on keeping control of a situation. You must learn to have trust and confidence in me. You should try to accept and act on these suggestions since they are for your benefit. In this way you can help yourself.

[The hypnotherapy then begins in earnest.]

T: We are deep in the basement now. As you step out of the elevator there is a passageway. This could be the passageway you saw the other day when you came to the bottom of the steps. Remember? I want you to walk down the passageway and describe to me exactly what you see.[1]

---

[1] Note how the therapist employs the structure provided by the patient in the first session and develops this content into a hypnoprojective exploration. In the hypnoprojective technique, the patient is stimulated to initiate a dreamlike

P: There are dark rooms. They are on both sides and the hall is dark. There is a light where I am.

T: I want you to choose a doorway.

P: The door on the left.

T: Step to the door and look in. As you look you will notice that the light surrounding you radiates into the room so that you can penetrate the darkness. Describe what the room is like.

P: I don't see anything yet. Just the window.

T: Walk to the window and look out. What's out there?

P: Sunshine, grass, trees.

T: Is this a scene you have viewed before? Do you know where you are?

P: It seems as if I have seen it but I don't know where.

T: As you turn around there is something there. What is it?

P: It looks like a hospital cart. There is nobody on it.

T: Who should be on it?

P: I don't know.

T: How do you feel about the room?

P: I don't feel comfortable.

T: There is something about the room that makes you feel uncomfortable? Do you want to leave?

P: I think so.

T: Shall we go out of the room now, back into the hall? [Pause.]

P: No, I am still in that room.

T: Something there interests you?

P: Just the hospital cart.

T: As you look at the hospital cart, a train of associations begins to come, ideas and feelings about the cart. You have seen it someplace before. Where have you seen this cart?

P: In the delivery room. I am lying on the cart.

T: When is this? What is the date today?

P: June.

T: *You* are lying there on the cart. It is June. What year?

The answer was either in June, 1947, or 1948, revealing the fact that the patient was in a delivery room in Jackson, Missis-

---

fantasy, care being exercised that the content elicited is not suggested or directed by the therapist; that is, the patient is encouraged to develop and respond to his own fantasy productions with continuing projective structuring so that he becomes immersed in an ongoing and, for him, exceedingly realistic fantasy situation (see Moss, 1957b).

sippi, in each year attempting to give birth to a male infant, neither of whom lived. Even though a number of hypnotic techniques were employed, they were unsuccessful in revealing the elusive verbalization made by her doctor. Through automatic writing, she did recapture the statement, "The baby is dead and she'll go too." Even though the patient had been under a general anesthetic, this procedure was based on the premise of the correctness of David Cheek's repeated observation that surgical patients are much aware of what goes on in the operating room. Dr. Cheek stresses the importance of recognizing that surgical patients behave under anesthetic as though they were actually hypnotized (1959, 1964).

T: We have been talking about memories which are distressing to you. We must see if you are ready to face up to them. You said you could stand considerable pain. Between now and when I see you next, your unconscious will select out the memory you have forgotten. This memory will push its way up so that when we meet and I put you under hypnosis we will be able to come in contact with the memory if you are strong enough and really want to remember what it is. Do you have anything to say now before I wake you up? [Patient nods negatively.] Now I want you to sleep deeply for a few minutes so that when you awaken you will feel happy and relaxed for having worked on your problem. When you do awaken you will have difficulty remembering what we talked about. It may also be best that for the next time or two that you come by yourself in case there is something you want to confide confidentially. [The patient is then awakened.]

P: [She asks immediately] Do you have a father in Urbana, Illinois, who is a doctor?

T: No, I don't, why do you ask?

P: There is a Dr. Moss there, an elderly gentleman. We were there when my husband got his last two degrees, 1940 to 1943.

T: How do you feel about this session today?

P: Fine, a little depressed but I don't know why.

T: Is it difficult to specifically remember what we talked about?

P: Yes.

T: I would suggest you don't recall it for a while.

P: Did you know Dr. Moss in Urbana? Maybe the old gentleman

died. He was quite elderly when we were there. It is funny I should think of him.[2]

Session III, January 31

P: It has been a *very* depressing week. A little humor was injected into the matter, however. My craft class started working in leather and the pounding almost put me to sleep. It sounded just like when you pound on the desk, and I was so sleepy I could hardly stay awake. We went to a dinner party and I think my husband was very embarrassed. I had great trouble staying awake during the concert afterwards in spite of a wonderful artist. Ordinarily, I would not have such trouble. But when I came home last night, I couldn't go to sleep and I never have trouble sleeping. So you will have to tell that little gimmick that only when *you* hit on the desk do I go to sleep. My class would be so amused if they knew that they almost put me to sleep.

T: What's been going on the last few days to make you feel so depressed?

P: I have been reliving things. You see, I wasn't smart enough to know that if I wanted to remember one thing I also had to remember all the things associated with it. So I have remembered things I haven't thought of in many years, and then last night when I couldn't sleep, I was trying to remember some little, sort of half-remembered thing. It was a scene in a hospital. A big room with lots of beds. I asked my husband this morning if he could remember anything like that connected with this incident I wanted to remember. He couldn't either but he has always kept a family diary which I never read. He is very methodical. I went through it this morning and found the incident I kept trying to remember. It wasn't terribly important. It was just part of the total scene.

T: At least you found some evidence that your memory was correct.

P: Yes, so I found out what it was and he had forgotten just as I had too. It was sort of like a jigsaw puzzle. I had to remember the pieces and put them all together. I guess I had not done all my homework so I had to stay awake last night and finish. I guess it is all straightened out now. It doesn't seem so important.

---

[2] Both references to the other Dr. Moss are obviously intruding thoughts as a result of the posthypnotic suggestion "not to remember." They provide an excuse not to remember and in that sense are similar to the rationalizations conveniently developed by subjects when called upon to explain their responses to posthypnotic suggestion.

T: You think you have all the pieces now?

P: I think so. Unless, does one's mind ever play tricks and place something else in place of what you are trying to remember?

T: Possibly.

P: I wondered about that when I tried to remember what was said in the delivery room. Something always comes back I had never thought of before, something very remote. The conversation part I knew is followed by something that was very remote, just like out of the sky and I can't understand it. The act of remembering seems more important than what I remember. It was so impressed on my mind that I had to remember and when I came out of the delivery room I couldn't. The feeling has lasted down through the years and it baffles me because I asked the nurse in Jackson what it was I wanted to remember because I knew she had heard it and she told me I shouldn't try to remember it. Of course, that was the wrong thing because I was determined to try to remember it. It wasn't that important, if only she had told me.

T: Do you want me to know what it was?

P: It doesn't matter. It was so simple it was silly. Many more things are so much more important. I had thought it was something to do with the baby's death and if it was I would like to know. I kept thinking something happened that was important. Apparently that was not so. It seems that it was a very rough day. Things did not progress as they should. I was in the delivery room from five in the morning until six in the evening. Sometime in the afternoon Dr. Wright came in and I asked him if he should do a section and he said it was too late. After that he said to the nurse, "Whenever you are ready, tell me." The thing I couldn't remember, it now seems, was his remark, "If we wait, she may go too." So it didn't refer to the baby at all as I thought it had. That was such a surprise to me I thought my mind was playing a trick on me but when I try to remember that is all I can think of.

When I talked to my husband he said that early in the morning the doctor had suggested a section and he asked him not to and he said he had blamed himself all these years. We had not discussed it all these years. I really think he was relieved when we talked about it. Then I talked to this nurse friend of mine of what we were doing here in these sessions. She said, having been a nurse in the delivery room, there might have been a short time of danger and if the doctor had gone on with the section I might not have survived. Since it was later diagnosed that I had pernicious anemia, I could have been in danger. Remembering this, if this is what it is, I think my husband feels a lot better about it. He carried a blame around I didn't know he had.

I thought I could look back at those two years sort of objectively but remembering this week it was really a pretty rough time. It is nice we do not remember for long. I am going to forget this, am I not? I don't want to recall all these things. It is so depressing.

T: What is it specifically that you recalled that was so depressing?

P: The baby's death and our wanting the child so badly. I had forgotten how hurt we both were. I am amazed that one can remember things so acutely. Time heals so well that you forget that the hurt is still there.

T: You can appreciate now how forgetting protects one.

P: Yes, I don't think one could carry all the hurts that one has in a lifetime. You would not have enough constitution for that.

T: This has been quite an experience for you.

P: Yes, and I wouldn't have missed it even though I was very depressed this week and had a hard time keeping my mind on other things. But I think it is encouraging, if I can remember this maybe I can remember about the dog.

T: If it is agreeable with you, let's explore this hospital scene once more in order to satisfy yourself that this was what actually happened.

P: Yes, I would like to be sure.

T: Then I will give you suggestions which will help you to store these memories away again. Is this acceptable to you?

P: Yes.

Hypnosis was rapidly induced by the tapping method. It was again suggested that she go deeper than before. The suggestion was made that she discriminate clearly between the hypnotic-inducing taps and similar sounds that she might hear outside the sessions. It was emphasized that the taps themselves were not sleep-producing. It was the meaning of the tapping in *this* particular situation and in *this* unique relationship with the therapist which caused them to be effective.

T: You have done excellently on your homework even though, quite naturally, you have been depressed by what you remembered. If it is agreeable to you we will look once more at this troublesome scene and then we will heal this old wound, and you will be able to forget about it in time. I told you last week that, if you wished, between sessions you would be able to completely remember what occurred at the time of your delivery. During that session you remembered much that had transpired, but some escaped you. I suggested that the specific memory you searched for would push up and you would remember as much as you could face. Apparently this has happened, and during the week many old memories returned until finally, last night, the climax arrived and you seemed to remember everything. I also told you that if there was something too painful to face, you did not have to. These same instructions remain in force. When I snap my fingers, any part that you have not yet recalled and which you can face will suddenly occur to you: just as you have had a name on the tip of your tongue and could not recall it and later when you relaxed the name spontaneously occurs. This is your final opportunity, if there is anything else that you wish to remember. If you do remember something additional which is disturbing, you have the option of remembering when you awaken or of burying it again. [The therapist then snaps his fingers. Patient's face contorts and she looks very distressed.]

T: Tell me now what came to mind.

P: "It's neck is broken."

T: This is apparently the thing that you wanted to remember?

P: Yes.

T: Had you thought of this recently?

P: No.

T: Do you think you knew it at some time previous?

P: I don't know.

T: Is there anything more to the situation to be recalled?

P: No, I think that is all.

T: This is a very tragic thing to happen. It must be painful recalling this now. You do want to remember this after you awaken?

P: Yes, I want to remember.

T: As I said before, you can see how memory through its distortions and omissions protects us from pain.

P: I don't think it could have been helped. I hope it couldn't have been helped.

T: It was a very unfortunate experience. Do you in any way blame yourself for what happened?

P: I don't think so. I don't think I blame anyone.

T: But apparently your husband carried some feeling of blame over the years. Do you think it is good that he finally got this out and talked about it?

P: I think so.

T: I think so too. I think this is part of the cleansing process. Sometimes things happen that no one could help. Having opened this wound, looked into it, probed and cleansed it with recall and in talking it over with your husband, do you think we can then close, sew it up, and forget about it? [The patient is then awakened.]

T: Do you remember what we talked about? Is there anything you would like to say about this experience?

P: [Reflectively] Why did it happen? It was especially tragic to us because it was our third loss. I guess we were supposed to adopt Judy and have a little girl. I was just thinking that maybe we had to lose the three in order to get Judy. I am glad we have her. She is a lovely girl and we could not choose between her and the three we lost, if we had to. She is a very sweet girl. She and her daddy are very close.

T: Do you think you and your husband will be any happier having faced up to the past?

P: We have always been very happy. I think this has been the one thing in our lives we could not talk about. We just didn't. We could talk about the years before and the years after, but those years we just could not talk about. They were unhappy years. I am sure he was as depressed as I but did not show it. I think it was upsetting enough that when faced with the decision to remain where we were or come here, we decided on the latter in order to get away from the situation in which we had had so much unhappiness. If he was carrying this blame, maybe he won't worry so much about it anymore, because he wasn't to blame. It was just something that could not be prevented. I think I sort of have the philosophy that if everyone's life is totaled against everyone else's, the outcome is about the same. There are just different types of sorrows in people's lives. Having lost three children, I have been much better able to understand other people's troubles and sympathize with them and help them.

T: Tragedy sharpens our sense of responsibility for other people.

P: I think it does. Maybe it was necessary. Who knows? We still have Judy. I didn't know until I was reading the family diary of some events surrounding this, on the day after this, this was on the 22nd of June, on the 23rd my husband again went to the Children's Home and talked to them about adoption. We had tried after having lost the little girl in 1947 and had started steps toward adoption. He went the next day after this happened, and almost all of the adoption steps were taken by him. I think I felt that a father must have to want to adopt a child a little more than a mother since maternal instincts might lead one astray. I have been quite happy that he took the steps toward adopting Judy, and they have been so mutually happy. Right now they are out sleigh-riding together. So life is not all dark. It has many bright spots.

T: There are certainly definite turning points in one's life, aren't there?

P: Very definitely. They color one's whole life. If these things had not happened, doubtless we would still be there in Mississippi. In forgetting the unpleasant things I had also forgotten how very many good friends we had who encouraged us. Of course, at the time, I was depressed and wished they had left me alone. I felt I had to reconcile myself to it alone. In the diary there was not a day that someone did not show us a kindness. Some of those people I had even forgotten. One should not forget how many friends we have when we are in trouble, but I guess it all had to be forgotten together.

T: It seems to be true that when we try to forget the unpleasant things that happen to us we also forget the positive things too. The mind is just not that precise in blotting out the past.

P: I thought I could just remember one little thing that had a mark around it and not remember everything, but maybe it was good to remember. Maybe I needed to be reminded there is still much to be thankful for.

T: Perhaps at the very least this will give you some new perspective on your present life, having had a chance to stand off from it and evaluate yourself again.

P: It can also make me understand why people sometimes do not get through things like this. I was very depressed. As I read the diary, there was day after day when my husband noted how discouraged I was. I did not think my husband had known how discouraged I felt. I had forgotten that I would take long walks at night by myself.

T: It must have been a very difficult time for you, but I would say at this point that you have done a good job of finally facing up to these feelings. [Long pause.] I wonder if you feel ready now to face your feelings about dogs.

P: Yes, I think I am.

T: It is difficult to imagine that it can be any more serious than you have told me about already.

P: Yes, I am sure it is the most tragic thing that has ever happened. This fear seems trivial now. I should be able to talk myself out of it but I can't.

T: During the past week you may have asked yourself how you got into the position of digging up the painful past.

P: No, I am glad I did. It seemed important that I remember.

T: I am glad you feel that way about it. I have confidence you will be able to handle the feelings we have brought up.

P: Yes, I believe so.

T: We do not have much time remaining this afternoon. If you will relax, I will begin your homework assignment.

P: All right, but have me do it in the daytime, if you can, rather than at night.

T: I will try not to make it as disturbing as it was before, just don't put the most unpleasant part off to the last moment.

P: Oddly enough, I did not mind. Perhaps I should not have tried to fill my mind with so many other things when it was trying so hard to remember. I even manufactured projects, projects I had lying around for a long, long time. I guess I thought I should try to keep my mind off it, but actually I was cheating myself. I won't do that this week.

T: [Small laugh.] Good. I hope the effect of the suggestions won't be quite so bothersome, at least not so distracting during the day.

P: I must get over it by Tuesday as that is Judy's birthday, and I want to give her a puppy.

T: That gives us something to aim for, doesn't it?

P: Yes, she keeps asking about the puppy. She is going to lose faith in you.

T: Actually you should be quite proud of yourself for being able to remember so much already.

P: Yes, if I could remember this, I surely can remember whatever happened to make me afraid of dogs. It does encourage me.

T: All right, now relax and here we go. [Taps desk. It is once again suggested that the patient go deeper than ever before.]

T: During this session and next I want the deepest part of your mind to begin to tell you about your fear of dogs — what this fear means and where it originated. The unconscious has difficulty speaking directly. Instead, it will speak in its natural language, dreams, so that in the next night or two you will have several very vivid dreams. Like most dreams you may not understand what they mean. Nevertheless, you will remember them completely and you will write them down to make certain you do not forget. Keep a pad of paper and a pencil by your bed, and in the morning, awaken gradually so as to recall the dream and be able to write it down in detail. As I said, they will appear to you as regular night dreams, but in these dreams your unconscious will convey to you, from the deepest sources of your memory, what your fear of dogs means and where this fear came from. You will bring these dreams in to our next session. Now, when you awaken, it will be as if from a very deep sleep and you will not recall the suggestion I have just given you. [The patient is awakened.]

P: [Immediately] You didn't contact my husband last week, did you? I thought maybe you might have.

T: No, why do you ask?

P: Both Wednesday and Thursday he didn't go back to the office. I thought perhaps he was asked to help keep my mind off of what I was trying to remember. He doesn't usually do that when he has things to do.

T: Did he want to come today?

P: I think he would have liked to have been invited along.

T: Why didn't you ask him?

P: I thought it might make him unhappy. I knew it was on tape and if he wanted to hear it later you would let him.

T: Yes, you can certainly tell him everything here has been recorded and he will be welcome to listen to it.

P: I did, but I thought his being here might make him unhappy because it made me unhappy, and I didn't want him to be unhappy.

T: Are you certain you want to tell him what we have talked about today?

P: Yes, I think so. We have always been very honest with each other.

T: The time is up for today. Incidentally, would you keep a pad of paper and pencil by your bed and if you happen to have any dreams, write them down? Do you dream very often?

P: No, I seldom dream.

T: Most people maintain they don't dream very frequently.

P: If I do, I don't remember them.

T: Well, will you please pay a little special attention for the next few nights and write them down for me?

Session IV, February 3

P: I kept my dreams. I did not dream Friday night, and I did not sleep much Saturday night because Judy was ill but I did have a dream. Do you want me to read them to you? This one was Saturday night. It was about two little girls, toddlers. It was a very disturbing dream, incidentally. One child was playing with the other as if she were a doll. She was carrying her, putting her face next to hers, but the one that was being carried around was dead. I went to sleep worrying about Judy so that might account for that. It seems as if the live one was my little girl and I was distressed when she picked up the dead one because she did not realize she was dead. I asked the undertaker what sort of embalming fluid he used and whether it would hurt my little girl. My concern seemed to be for her. Then there was something about redressing the dead baby and I was concerned about this. The undertaker or somebody was dressing it on a bed and I was very sad because it was so still, and then it seemed as if I was trying to get a box of a specific size but I could not remember what the size was. I guess I needed the big box to put the little ones in. It seemed like I needed them for clothes or toys or something. And then it seemed as if I were at my sewing machine mending a badly torn dress. Suddenly I realized my child was dead and I cried a lot in my dream. Then it seemed there was only one child, the dead one, and it was mine. It was a very sad and depressing dream. I never had a dream like that before. It was horrible even when I thought of it in the daytime. And I didn't have anything to drink before I went to bed.

Sunday night I had a vague dream but as I recorded it, it seemed to come back. It was something about wanting to get flowers to plant and Judy was with me. We were visiting some friends on a grassy hill. I left to go back to my car. It was an old car, but not a car I had ever seen in my lifetime. Some people went back to the car with me. I expected Judy to follow but she didn't. I went back to find her in the crowd but could not and I was quite angry with her for not coming with me. While looking for her I saw some people using stones to build a formal garden. It was pretty and I was interested in it. They had lots of flowers, bronze chrysanthemums. I asked where they got them and they said a playground down the

road was being torn up for a building site and there might be
enough flowers so that I could get flowers to plant if I wanted
them. They were making a flower garden and I was amused because they said a filling station would be there and that was funny
because it did not look like it would be a filling station. It looked
like it would be a flower garden. And I was very sorry that I had
been angry with Judy for I realized she was little and probably
could not find her way in the crowd. I do not know if I ever found
her or not, but I was sorry when I woke up that I had been angry
with her.

T: It didn't seem fair to blame her when she was so small. Were you
surprised at having these dreams and being able to remember
them?

P: No, but I was surprised that the one was so horrible. I wasn't
surprised to remember them because you had told me to write
them down. At first when I did go to record them they would be
rather vague, but as I wrote them down they would come to me.[3]

T: This matter of digging up the past can be very painful, can't it?

P: Yes, and oddly enough when I woke from that horrible dream, I
recalled my little sister's death and I haven't thought of that for
many, many years. I recall practically nothing about it. It is so long
ago I just never think about that.

T: How long ago was this?

P: Well, if I tell you the truth I will be telling you my age and a
woman should never do that. It must have been about 41 years
ago, I was about four. I was too small to recall much about it.
Just two or three things I have remembered through the years.

T: Somehow this dream restimulated the memory?

P: I don't know because I have not thought about that for many,
many years. But I thought of that and I thought it might be important so I wrote it down too. There are only about two or three
things I remember about it. I recall one of the older ladies said,
"Let her go in there and see her if she wants to," or something like
that. I do remember wanting to go and view my sister. She was
younger, about two, I guess. But I don't remember much else
about it. One thing of interest through the years to me is how children can misinterpret what adults say to them. One of the elderly
ladies in the neighborhood said that my sister had gone away and

---

[3] Noteworthy is the patient's complete faith in the instruction that she would be
able to recall her dream. Also characteristic of the posthypnotic suggesion is the
spontaneous improvement in memory as she initiated the act of recall.

tried to describe heaven to me. What that put in my mind was that she was way far away and very high up. That was all that was implanted in my mind. The following year, my folks moved away from the little country town to St. Louis and I was quite happy, because I thought it was a long distance and I would see my sister. I was even happier when we got off at the Tower Grove station and went up that long flight of stairs. I thought my little sister would be up there. But of course she wasn't, and I thought, "Those ladies, they foxed me!" That taught me when I got older that you must be very careful what you say to a child. They often do not understand.

T: Do either of these dreams have any meaning to you?

P: No, Judy was definitely in one but they do not mean anything to me.

T: Would you like to explore into their meaning?

P: Yes, but I kept hoping I would not have to go into the horrible dream. It was so horrible that it frightened me. I don't know why it seemed so horrible.

T: It is up to you.

P: I think everybody feels that sometimes you want to and sometimes you don't, but I want to get through this thing. When I clean house I clean out all the corners. I really do want to get through with it. If it has something to do with it, I want to find out what.

T: I think you can understand that very often the things that patients are most reluctant to explore are the very things which are most closely related to their difficulties.

P: Yes, I know that.

T: It is possible that this dream which is so horrible to you may provide some key to your problem.

P: Yes, but I don't know how. The only thing similar in my life was my sister's death, but I don't know why that should upset me.

T: But it is odd that you should have this particular memory upon awakening from the dream.

P: Yes, and I thought about it in such a fearful way. I had really expected to find my two "ornery" brothers siccing their dog on me, but maybe I won't find that.

T: If you think you can stand up to this we can begin.

P: [Resolutely] I can stand up to anything, I hope.

T: You have undergone a lot of pain in your life. I have confidence that you will be able to face this. After all, this memory you relate happened over 40 years ago. What you seem to be doing is perhaps reacting to it as you did as a little girl. If this dream and memory are associated with your fear of dogs, as we were talking about it the other day, here, too, you seem to be reacting as a little girl rather than as a grown-up.

P: Yes, and I am still afraid of dogs. Saturday when we were out, there were dogs yapping about and I was obviously afraid. My husband laughed and said to the puppies, "Come back next week and she will be friendlier." But I was afraid. Going into class the other morning we met five or six dogs and I thought, "Which of these dogs am I most afraid of?" I was not afraid of the big one at all. The little frisky one I was. I don't know what I was afraid of but I act just like a child when they come around. I know an adult should not act that way but I can't help it.

T: You still retain a child's feelings about dogs. Then perhaps the answer lies somewhere back in your childhood?

P: It *must* since I have had it all my life. You would laugh to know how many dinner invitations I have turned down because I thought they had a dog in the house. That is as abnormal as it can be, isn't it? Don't answer because I know it is.

T: There are actually many people who have something specific they are unaccountably afraid of.

P: The only encouraging thing is when the minister said the other day that he has yet to meet a normal person. I know it is abnormal and I would like very much to get rid of it.

T: Well, let us see if you are willing to pay the price.

P: I think it would be worth anything, I really do.

[Hypnosis is induced by the tapping method.]

T: I told you at our last meeting that you would have dreams related to your fear of dogs. And you apparently complied very nicely: you brought in two dreams, even though the first made you highly anxious. You have affirmed your resolution to face up to this thing even if you find it temporarily painful. You have already demonstrated in the last session your ability to face up to painful past experiences.

Now we have another memory to uncover, with the possibility that when you recover it, talk about it, and live with it, you will find that after all these years you may be able to establish control of this fear that bothers you. I am very interested in the dream you had Saturday night and I think we should examine it carefully. You seem to have done a faithful job recording it. In order to assure ourselves that you have not forgotten any of it, however, I want you to try to experience the dream again. Since it was intensely painful, I am going to help you remove yourself from the dream. Rather than having you actually re-experience the dream, I want you to return to our movie theater. Remember the movie theater? I want you to seat yourself. Only you and I are there. Remember that I am there beside you. In a moment I will snap my fingers. When I do you will see a movie of the dream you had Saturday night. You will see it just as it happened in every detail. When the movie begins you will please signal [by raising a finger]. When it is completed I want you to signal again. Then I want you to tell me about it exactly as you saw it. Do you understand?

P: Yes.

T: The projectionist is getting ready. In a moment you will see the movie. It will be clear and vivid but less disturbing because you will always remember you are sitting in the movie theater only looking at the screen. Do you understand?

P: Yes.

T: All right, you are looking at the blank screen and here comes the picture. [After a pause of 45 seconds in which the patient makes no response] Do you see the movie screen?

P: Yes.

T: Is there a movie on it?

P: No.

T: Why not?

P: I am afraid.

T: Can you face this? It is up to you.

P: I want to face it.

T: Now you are in the movie theater, *I* am sitting there close beside you. In a moment, if you really want to find out the meaning of the dream, the movie will begin. When you are ready the projectionist will begin the film.

[After a 30-second lapse the patient signals that the "movie" has begun. The patient looks obviously preoccupied and somewhat disturbed. Five minutes and 10 seconds elapse.]

T: Is it through now?

P: No.

T: Can you see it clearly?

P: Not very.

T: All right, tell me what you have experienced.

P: There was a room. There are two children. One is carrying the other and then my mother came. It does not look like my mother but it is my mother and she told me to put the baby down and I did. And then my mother and my father seem to be tired or ill or something. They are in the bed in the next room. Someone is changing the clothes and I found the big box that I could not find before [in the nocturnal dream] and they put the baby in the box. My mother told me I should not touch the box. I can look but I cannot touch. I don't want to touch the box. Then it is kind of hazy and that is all I know.[4]

T: What is it that you have been telling me here?

P: I guess it happened to me. It was that dress, it was torn.

T: Whose dress was it?

P: The baby's. It was torn.

T: How did it get torn?

P: I don't know how it got torn. It got torn. I don't know whether I tore it or someone else tore it.

T: Where did you see the dress?

P: After it was torn. After it wasn't on the baby. I don't know.

T: Listen to me. Is there more to this?

P: Well, there seems to be a little black dog but I don't know for sure that there is. If there is, I am not afraid of it. I don't know but there seems to be.

T: A little black dog?

P: Yes, with curly black hair but I am not afraid of it, because it is in that room too, and I don't feel afraid of it.

T: Listen carefully to me. You know that sometimes fortune tellers employ a crystal ball and claim to see the future in it. I don't know about that but I do know that in looking into a crystal ball you find it easy to see things in yourself, such as forgotten memories and experiences. I want you to look now into a crystal ball. You are in a darkened room. There are dark drapes on all sides except in the middle of the room there is a luminescent crystal ball. Can you see it?

P: Yes, I can see it.

T: There is the crystal ball. Go seat yourself before it. You see it clearly. I want you to sit and stare at the crystal ball and as you

[4] It becomes apparent here and in subsequent verbalizations that the patient had not re-experienced her dream, but instead, repressed fragmented memories associated with the early trauma are expressed. Her reaction of horror indicates its transparent nature — there is little condensation and no protective symbolization. Disguise is largely through omission of key fragments rather than distortion per se, e.g., the absence of any direct reference to the dog.

stare added details of the thing you have been telling me about will appear. Pictures from the past, pictures concerned with what was happening there in that room. Pictures concerned with your little sister and your relationship to her and also to the little black dog. As you stare, describe to me the things that appear to you.

P: My Aunt Ethel is standing there. [Moans.] My little sister and I are playing. There is a little dog there. My little sister is pretty. There is a woodpile. [Moans again.] My brothers are there too. They are carrying wood. My little sister has some pieces of wood in her hands. I don't have any. There is that same little dog.

T: Whose little dog is it?

P: I don't know, but it is staying with me.

T: It must have a name of some sort. All little dogs do.

P: I don't know it.

T: Listen carefully, maybe you can hear someone call it by name.

P: My mother is in the door; she is calling the little dog "Rover." It is going to her.

T: That must be its name then.[5]

P: [Moans.] It knocked my little sister over. [Plaintively] She fell on the wood.

T: Your little sister fell on the wood?

P: The wood she had in her hands. She is all right.

T: It didn't really hurt her?

P: I guess not. Mother took her into the house, then I went into the house. We are in the house now.

T: Tell me about the house and what is going on now.

P: Mother is looking at her face. Velma, that is her name. She is bleeding on the cheek.

T: She has a scratch?

P: She has a scratch. That seems to be all.

T: Now as you continue staring intently in the crystal ball you will find still other pictures, relating to your life there with the family, the little black dog, and your little sister. Down in the depths of the ball you see pictures forming; they seem to grow in size and float up to the top. What do you see now?

P: [Sighs deeply.] Well, there is a door from the room that leads onto the back porch. My mother thinks I knocked my sister over. They are going to play a little game. My brothers, big sister, and I are going to walk to the door. When the one who knocked her over

[5] Therapist intrudes on the patient's flow of associations in an attempt to elicit additional detail and facilitate memory, but the patient persists in her line of thought.

reaches the door, something will knock. When I get to the door something knocks, but I did not push my little sister over!

T: What happens now?

P: When I go to the door something knocks. I did not knock her over! But everybody thinks I did. They don't believe me when I tell them. I didn't hurt her!

T: Was it there in the yard they thought you knocked her over?

P: Yes, when she was running with the wood.

T: Actually, it was the little dog?

P: Yes, the little dog was playing with her. I was just watching.

T: They thought you did it?

P: Yes, but I didn't. It seems that this is all there is to this part.

T: But there must be more. What did they do to you because they think you pushed your sister over? Look there in the crystal ball. What did they do to you because of that?

P: I guess my mother is spanking me. I am on her lap and she is spanking me. Everybody watches.

T: How do you feel?

P: I don't like it because I didn't do it. I don't mind being spanked if I did something, but I didn't.

T: So you are being punished for something you didn't do.

P: I am in my own bed now.

T: What are you thinking there in your bed?

P: I wish they knew I didn't do it.

T: You feel badly?

P: [Sadly] I am unhappy.

T: Just keep talking about this and what happens next. As you look there in the ball the feelings, the memories, everything comes alive almost as if it were happening now.

P: My big sister is there. I am sleeping in her bed. She is comforting me. She doesn't think I did it. I don't think she thinks I did it. She was always my friend. Now it is morning, I guess. It is sort of cold in the house. It is breakfast time but I am not going to eat because I don't feel good. They blame me. I am unhappy about it.

T: It seems so unfair.

P: It seems like I am in the yard again, and the dog is in the yard with me.

T: This is the next day?

P: Yes, we are out by the woodpile again and I feel quite badly because they think I pushed my sister over, but I didn't, and my little sister is not out playing with me. She is ill. Dr. Donahue is coming. That is Dr. Donahue coming now. Then there are a lot of people there. My mother seems to be crying and my dad too. My little sister just looks like she is sleeping. She is awfully pretty.

T: Where is she?

P: She is lying on a bed. No, it is not a bed, it looks like an ironing board. Oh, I am looking for something and I find it now. It is a necklace. It is mine. I ask my Aunt Ethel to put it on her because it will look pretty on her, and my Aunt Ethel does. She looks awfully pretty. Now everybody is in the parlor and then Gordon comes in and they all start crying again.

T: Who is Gordon?

P: He was my sister's husband, but they were not married then. Helen always liked him. He goes in and sees her. She looks awfully pretty, and I go too. Then we come out in the parlor and he takes my hand. He likes us both. Then I go back in by myself. She looks so pretty lying there, so I think I will pick her up. She does not hug me like she usually does, though. I am holding her and the dog is with me. He wants to see her too. Oh, he tore her dress!

T: Pardon?

P: The dog, he tore her dress.

T: How did he do that?

P: He was jumping up on her and tore her dress, and Mother will not like that. The dog should not be in the house, but I do not think I let him in. I know I should put her down but I want to hold her.

T: What do you think and feel about her?

P: She is so pretty and so sweet. I just want to hold her.

T: What happens next?

P: My mother comes into the room. She is mad at me. She told me I should know better. Somebody took the baby away from me.

T: Did you want to give her up?

P: No, I wanted to hold her. It must be my Aunt Anna. She said I should not have torn her dress, but I didn't tear her dress.

T: [Simulating the mother] Somebody did. Who did it?

P: I didn't do it. Rover did it, I didn't. He didn't mean to, he just wanted to see her. Why doesn't that place on her face go away?

T: Rover tore her dress? She still has a scratch?

P: Oh, yes. It looks like a splinter in it. But Aunt Anna will fix it. She will change her dress and then it will be all right. She will put the necklace back on her, and now it is all right.

T: She has a new dress and the necklace on her?

P: Yes, a new dress and necklace and a bracelet on her arm. I think that is mine too. Yes, I want her to have it. Now they are going to put her in that box. I must not touch the box, but I can look over her if someone is with me.

I guess we are going somewhere now. Oh yes, we are going. [Sighs very deeply.]

T: Going where?

P: Going behind Aunt Mary's house to the cemetery. They are putting the box down in the ground. We are singing some kind of songs. I wish I could see her again, but I guess I won't.

T: Your little sister is gone now?

P: Yes, now it seems like it is some days later. I am on the back porch by myself. I wish she would come play with me. Mother comes out the back door and she sees me crying. I don't want her to see me crying.

T: You don't want her to know how you feel?

P: No, she thinks I hurt her but I didn't.

T: Your mother blames you for what happened to your sister?

P: She thinks I pushed her over. But I didn't. I don't seem to like my dog anymore.

T: He still wants to be friendly, doesn't he?

P: I don't want to be friends.

T: You don't like your little dog?

P: No, I don't like my little dog anymore. I want my sister.

T: Your little dog took your sister away from you?

P: I don't like him. I wish that they would take *him* away.

T: You want him to go away and your little sister to come back?

P: Yes.

T: Go on.

P: I am just lonely.

T: You are very lonely after your sister is gone?

P: Yes.

T: And unhappy because your mother blames you? You don't like your dog anymore?

P: No.

T: This feeling must go on for quite a while, doesn't it?

P: I guess so.

T: Now look into the crystal ball again. Other thoughts and feelings are coming to mind about what happened. Your feelings about your sister, your feelings about your mother, your feelings about yourself, and your feelings about Rover.

P: I wish she would give me to my Aunt Ethel. She nearly did.

T: You were so unhappy you wanted to be away from your mother?

P: I guess so. She nearly gave me to her when I was born, because she nearly died and they said she should give me to somebody. She gave me to my Aunt Ethel but she lived. Now I wish my Aunt Ethel had me. She doesn't blame me, she knows I didn't do that.

T: Does your mother keep reminding you?

P: [Sighs.] When I tell her I miss Velma she says it is my fault. I tell her it is not my fault.

T: When you tell her how you miss your little sister, she says it is your fault she is gone?

P: It is not my fault!

T: How does it make you feel?

P: I am *so* unhappy. She should see it is not my fault, Rover pushed her over.

T: Didn't you tell her this?

P: She doesn't believe me. Nobody believes me. Maybe my big sister does. I guess she does, but my mother doesn't.

T: How about your father?

P: I don't know about Dad.

T: How about your brothers?

P: I don't know about them.

T: It is mainly your mother who blames you? She makes you feel very unhappy.

P: She is lonely too, though.

T: How do you feel during this time about Rover?

P: I don't much want to play with him anymore.

T: How do you feel about him?

P: I don't like him anymore. He pushed her over. He tore her dress.

T: He pushed her over, tore her dress, and got your mother angry at you? So he is to blame for all this, yet *you* got punished.

P: I wish they would take him to my grandfather's farm.

T: You wish they would take him away. Does he remind you of what happened?

P: Yes.

T: What finally happens to Rover?

P: I guess he goes to Grandfather's farm.

T: And what happens to you?

P: I have to stay there.

T: You cannot go away?

P: I wish I could go to Aunt Ethel's.

T: You would be happier away from your mother?

P: Yes.

T: Any other pictures come to your mind?

P: It seems as if I have some flowers in my hand and I am going up back of Aunt Ethel's house. I have to hurry because if Mother catches me she won't like it. But Aunt Ethel sees me. She goes with me and that is better. She helps me plant them; then we come back down the hill together in the lane. I tell her goodbye but she thinks she had better go with me. She takes me home.

T: Does she tell your mother where you have been?

P: No.

T: Aunt Ethel understands, doesn't she?

P: Yes.

T: Time is growing short here this afternoon. I think it might be wise if we turn your attention to the second dream, if that is all right with you.

P: It is all right.

T: The essence of the dream seems to be that you witnessed a group of people building a formal garden. Judy became lost from you in the crowd and later you felt sorry that you had been angry at her. Look into the crystal ball. What is the relationship of this dream to what you have been telling me? As you look the meaning of this dream will occur piece by piece, like pieces of a jigsaw puzzle. Pictures are beginning to form. They are growing clearer. There is a picture, tell me about it.

P: That is a scene at Laural Hill Cemetery in St. Louis. There are men down there building some pretty fences. It seems, that is funny, it seems as if there are a lot of people going up there. I guess that is my older sister's death. Yes, that is my older sister. They are burying her there in that cemetery.

T: Other pictures are appearing one after another clearly so that you can understand piece by piece what the dream meant to you.

P: Oh, the filling station. That is when we were coming from Carbondale to St. Louis in the funeral procession. We stopped to get gas. My brother-in-law got a Coke. It seemed odd. I guess he didn't even think. We are back in the cemetery. They are burying my sister.

T: In the dream Judy became separated and you could not find her and you were very sorry you had been angry with her. What does that mean now?

P: I don't know.

T: Look in the crystal ball. There are other pictures forming which may tell you the meaning of that part of your dream.

P: My sister-in-law said I should have come down for the operation rather than her; but I was going to go take care of my sister. I would have gone but we did not expect her to die. I was going to take care of her.

T: Your sister-in-law thought you had neglected your duty?

P: She thought I should have been there for the operation.

T: You had no way of knowing she was going to die?

P: No, I was going to take care of her.

T: You felt badly when she died?

P: I saw her die, but I wasn't there for the operation.

T: What does it mean that you were sorry — that you were angry with Judy?

P: I don't know because I wasn't angry with anybody. Judy wasn't there at the time. I don't understand.

T: In a moment I will snap my fingers; you will have a second dream which means the same as the dream you had Sunday night except it will be clearer and easier to understand. The dream is slowly beginning to form. A dream that has the same meaning but is perhaps a little more direct. Are you ready for it now? [Snaps fingers.]

P: [After several minutes' pause] It is not clear.

T: Tell me what you have been thinking about.

P: I have been thinking about the dream. I have been thinking about what it means. I don't understand it.

T: Our time is almost up for this afternoon. I think we have made considerable progress this afternoon understanding your fear of little dogs.

There may be more, however, that we should know. You will find that as we recover these memories, your fear of dogs will naturally, gradually, decrease. It has become easy to see how you would have such intense feelings about dogs from what you have told me thus far. Again between sessions you will have one or more dreams, clearly experienced and remembered, concerning your fear of dogs. In another session or two we should have a very clear understanding of how this fear arose and how it grew. I want you to also have another dream which means the same as the one you had on Sunday night about the cemetery. Are there any additional questions you want to bring up at this time?

P: I don't think so.

T: Have we covered everything you want to talk about now?

P: I cannot think of anything else.

T: Sleep deeply for several minutes; then it will be as if you awakened from a deep sleep. You will remember only as much of what we have talked about as you can face.

[Instructions preparatory to awakening:] We have talked about your little sister's death and how distressed you were. The way in which it came about and the fact that you were blamed for it must have been very disturbing. It would have been to any child. Nevertheless, you are facing these memories as you never faced them since you grew up. You can face them now since it happened many years ago and you recognize that you cannot blame yourself.

In the next few days the pieces will unconsciously fall in place. You will come to an understanding of your concern about death and your relationship to death — what it meant to you when your little sister died, what it meant when your big sister died, what it meant when your three babies died. All of these events fall into a pattern. I don't want these meanings to come clearly to the surface until the next session when I will be with you to help you. At that time all of the pieces will well up and fit into place. Remember, I don't want this to occur until you return next time. Your unconscious, meantime, will prepare you to face all this. When you do face it, you will then fully recognize that your fear of dogs is only a symptom of the whole problem, and you will begin to lose your concern about them. Your fear of dogs is no more the real problem than the spots are in measles. Next time, if you are ready, we will face all these things, bring them out, talk about them, and put everything in its place. I think you have made real progress and have been a very good patient. You have shown real courage in facing up to these fears. Now, when I awaken you, you will remember as much as you can tolerate. You are free to remember or to forget.

P: [Stretches.] This is better than I have slept the last two nights. [Looks off into space reflectively.]

T: Can you tell me what you are thinking about?

P: I was thinking Mother *should* have been angry with me. I should not have picked up the baby but I didn't know. I should not have done that, should I? It must have shocked her terribly.[6]

---

[6] Note that the patient responded in such a manner as to rationalize and justify the mother's behavior rather than expressing resentment and hostility. She continues in this vein throughout the remainder of the session, reflecting a well-established habit of intrapunitiveness.

T: You can understand now how your mother must have felt.

P: Oh, yes, she must have felt terrible.

T: Did you know that your mother had blamed you?

P: Oh, no. Nobody ever mentioned that to me. I *didn't* know it. I never knew it happened in my conscious life at least.

T: Isn't it interesting how all of these details of our lives are stored away? Did you remember the dog jumping up?

P: Oh, no. I don't ever remember having a dog.

T: Do you remember now?

P: Yes.

T: What was his name?

P: Rover. Perhaps he is the little rascal in the picture that they were holding. [In the first session she remarked that there was a photograph taken of herself at a very young age in which she was seated next to a dog held by her two brothers.]

T: How sure are you that you had this dog?

P: I can't prove it but it just seems so. I guess Mother could tell me.

T: It would be interesting to check some of this with her.

P: I would like to know.

T: I think you should do that.

P: I would like to. My mother is an invalid in St. Louis. She lived with us for about a year and a half after Dad's death but it never worked out. She seemed to resent Judy. We didn't realize it was building up until the kindergarten teacher noticed it was causing Judy some difficulty so we had to change that arrangement. I will just have to go to St. Louis and see her. She could tell me a lot of these things. I guess she would, unless it was so horrible to her she wouldn't want to talk about it. There is no one else. If my dad were living I could talk to him. I could talk to him about anything.

T: How about your brothers?

P: The one brother I could talk to best is in California; the other is in St. Louis but we have never been close.

T: Did you ever suspect that your mother had blamed you?

P: Oh, no, I didn't know Mother had blamed me. I can understand, though, some of my actions as a child. I always wanted to please everybody. I can remember that at school I would take blame for things that other kids did and my mother would get real provoked with me because every week she had to go to the principal. If the teacher wanted to blame somebody I was always glad to take the blame. As I grew older I realized it was real stupid but I guess I didn't want to be blamed for anything, I mean I didn't want anybody to be blamed for anything, so I took the blame. I was mixed up, I know that. I wanted people to like me as a child. I expect that Mother must have been terribly upset about me picking up the baby. Of course, if she believed I had caused her to fall she would have blamed me.

T: Did you consciously recall your little sister's death?

P: I remembered very little about it. I remember she died. I heard them talk about it. The doctor in this little town didn't know what was the matter. They removed a splinter from her face. He thought it was an infection perhaps but I didn't know what had happened.

T: Do you think your mother would admit to you how she had felt?

P: I doubt it.

T: It might be a very sensitive point.

P: I think so. I wouldn't want to ask her *that* but I would like to ask her about some details. It is rather hopeless — she didn't know the dog pushed Velma.

T: But she would probably remember the incident in the yard.

P: She surely would. Anything as important as that. Do you think she would remember my picking up the baby?

T: Or the torn dress?

P: Yes, that must have horrified her. I know it did because when I had the dream, I shuddered to think that Judy would do a thing like that.

T: You put yourself in your mother's place in the dream, didn't you?

P: I guess I did. I wonder why.

T: It was Judy instead of you.

P: Yes, I was concerned about Judy doing it though it didn't seem to be Judy in the first dream. There were just two children. The one doing the picking up seemed to be mine or me. It doesn't seem as bad now as it did yesterday. It just seems like, like an incident. It must have been very shocking to my mother. I would like to know if she remembers any of these things.

T: There are a lot of details you recalled here you might mention to her.

P: Yes, it is funny I should have thought about my older sister's death. That would not be connected with it in any way, would it? I had this fear so much longer ago than that.

T: Let your unconscious work on that problem for a little while, shall we?

P: I guess so.

T: You may notice that through these sessions runs a theme about death.

P: Yes, I had noticed that but I don't think I feel unkindly toward death. It is something I have thought a lot about and talked to people about. I think a turning point in my thinking about death was after my older sister's death. If I had been afraid of it before, I wasn't afraid of it anymore, because she was the best person I had ever known — a very good person, a minister's wife, and did more for everybody than most anybody I ever knew. Her death seemed so unnecessary. She was only 39. Seeing her die, I felt differently about death. It no longer seemed mysterious, something one might feel curious about but not fear. I have been thankful I was there to see her die since it gave me a different attitude.

T: Maybe you are already beginning to answer some of the questions of the relationship here between the death of your younger sister and that of your older sister. Let's leave that go until we meet again. When do you want to meet again? I think a few more sessions may be sufficient.

Session V, February 6

P: If there is any question about our making progress, we are. Tuesday morning when I went to class I wished I would meet a dog. I was curious as to how I would react. It must have been the first morning in weeks that I didn't meet a dog. But in coming back from class I met a big Collie. I thought, "I am going to pet him." And I felt differently towards a dog than I have ever felt. Is it possible to feel sorry for a dog? That is the way I felt. I was able to stroke his fur and pet him. I was doing real well until the Smith's dog saw what was happening. I guess he was so amazed at seeing me pet one of his friends that he decided that he would run over too. When I saw him coming I started saying, "Go away, go away." The same old thing. But I think we have made progress. I think that is the first time I ever willingly petted a dog.

Of course, I was quite taken aback by what we discovered last time. I didn't know whether my mind was making it up or if it really happened. I went home and talked to my husband immediately about it and it all made sense to him. He had observed my family and me and it was obvious to him that they seemed to feel that I owed them something. I never felt that way especially. I knew that if they needed help they always asked me, and I was always in a

position to help them. I didn't have children and my sister did. I
said that if they really felt that I was to blame for that loss back
there they unconsciously might feel that I owed them something.

T: They acted as if you had some moral obligation to them?

P: Yes, my husband says so, though I never particularly felt that they
acted that way. But I thought that if it made sense to him it must
really have happened. I guess that is why I have worked so hard
this week. These things that I remembered, I had to find some
proof they actually happened. So I kept digging to see if I could
find evidence they really did.

On Monday night I seemed to dream a lot but I was unable to
recall anything except something about a shoe box and a head of
cabbage in it. That isn't much to go on.

Tuesday was a worse day than any I have had so far. The depression was more intense than it has been at any time. It was so
emphatic that all day long I could not shake it. One thing that was
rather interesting to me, Judy was slightly ill and stayed at home
playing around the house. I thought I would do a quick pencil
sketch of her. She is a very happy child, her whole face radiates
happiness, but I could not catch it. Every sketch that I made had
a sad face. I guess I couldn't shake off my own feelings enough to
catch her appearance. I think I will keep the one sketch even
though it has a very sad face.

T: This feeling was very pervasive. I would like to see the sketch too.

P: At first I felt, "This is nothing I want to keep," but I know there
is still one and I will bring it. But I couldn't get away from that
feeling. Tuesday night was real rough. When I went to bed I
couldn't get to sleep. That is not too normal. Usually I read and
fall asleep but I couldn't get to sleep. I dreamed about several
people but when I awakened from it, it was too vague to recall. I
kept thinking about so many things that I had to get up and record
them. I thought of them once and I thought of them in the same
sequence again so I wrote them down.

When I woke up I found myself thinking about the loss of our first
child in 1943 and my dad's death in 1953. I can see no connection
between those things at all. I just thought of them as incidents and
not as anything depressing. Then I recalled an incident in October,
1943, when I could not get my car out of the garage. My husband
finished his degree in June at the University of Illinois; two days
before he got his doctorate, he got inducted in the Army. I went

home to my folks. There wasn't much else to do. I remember one time in October my car was in the garage near Dad's store and I couldn't get it out. I was irked when Dad didn't come out of the store to help me. I should not have been irked because in the first place my dad could not drive and could not have helped anyhow. I don't know what I expected him to do — move the garage, I guess. So I went back to the garage and got it out but, like a woman, tore the facing off the garage door. Uncle Jud fixed it. I wanted to visit Charles, my husband's brother, and his daughter. I recall the feeling of being sad and lonely being away from my husband. A few days after that we lost the first child.

Then I wrote here that I recalled teasing my husband's mother about what I would do if he ever left me. That was an amusing thing. Some young girl had left her husband and went back to her mother. I remember kidding her about what I would do if my husband left me, since I always felt more at home there than I did with my own family and she knew it. She laughed and said, "Don't you worry about Preston, you just come on home." It was an amusing thing, but for some reason I seem to recall that.

And then I recalled the summer of 1939. I finished college that year and Preston was beginning work at Illinois. I stayed at home that summer working in Dad's store. He needed the help. We were very poor then and it was the best arrangement. I was unhappy because Dad objected to the brother of the groceryman across the street spending so much time talking to me. I had not even remembered that event so I had to find out. It was vague, something about playing golf and I was irked at my dad's objections. The young man seemed nice and I knew Preston would understand. I think I have mentioned that my husband is very methodical in everything he does. He has kept every letter we ever wrote to each other in chronological order. I had the date put down in my mind so all I had to do was go upstairs and look in the trunk and, yes, it was there. He was a young St. Louis University student, a Catholic boy, a history major. In the neighborhood where I grew up very few people had gone on to school so we had something in common, and it was very natural for us and there was nothing wrong for the young man to walk home with me or come down to our parlor to study with me. I remember I was very irked with Dad, but now looking at it from a more mature angle I can see his point of view. Of course, it was a very innocent thing. About the golf clubs, I asked Preston in the letter if he would like to buy some golf clubs that this young man had, an extra set that he wanted to sell. Now it strikes me as a humorous note. I think he could have bought the whole set for $5. This year at Christmas my husband gave me a set of golf clubs. If he had known this before we could probably have saved some money. So that actually happened and I have proof of that.

Then I recalled my last year of college. Each memory I had goes back a little further. The memory I just told you about was after I graduated. Now this is the last year in college. I read Lin Yutang's *Importance of Living* three times. Apparently I liked it. I don't remember that I read *Gone with the Wind* three times so I decided I would have to find out why I liked that book so well. At the coffee hour this morning there were several professors there and I was talking to them about this book. I asked if they were familiar with the book and knew why I had read it so many times. Dr. Roberts said perhaps it was because the author used such beautiful, chaste English. That did not quite satisfy me. It may have been that, but I don't think it would make me read the book three times. Dr. Nichols thought that maybe it was his manner of presentation. But that did not satisfy me either so I had to find the book and I did, and I am going to read it and find out why I read it three times. There must have been a reason, especially because I recall we were both working very hard at the time.

Another thing that came to mind though I wasn't sure that it happened: it seemed important that I remember that I graduated with honors. I could not remember that I had. It wasn't that important to me then. I asked my husband and he could not remember it. The thing that was most important to us then about graduation was getting the ceremony over and getting on to other things in our life. We found my diploma but I could not find anything to indicate that I had graduated with honors. I did find my transcription and added up the grades and my husband said, well, yes, it looked as if I had. So I guess my mind did not make that up but it seems to be important to me to know if all these things actually happened because I was a little skeptical that this other could have happened. But everything I have been able to check proved out.

T: It is difficult for you to believe that you could have forgotten something as important as this?

P: I believe so. It seems as if I would have remembered something about it.

After that I remembered something that seems rather important now, but I did not know that it was at the time. I felt disappointed that none of my family came to my graduation. I recall giving my tickets to some strangers. My husband was on the platform with the rest of the faculty so I did not have anyone out front. It did not seem important to me then but I must have thought a lot about it in order for it to make this impression. In the first place they had objected to my going to school. They thought I was wasting my money. It was not that they objected to spending their money because I worked my way through without any financial assistance from them. I worked two years and ran out of funds so then Preston and I got married so I could go on to school. Of course, we had been engaged three years before that.

Then I was back further in my life to a surprise birthday party I gave to myself. My mother was very displeased. I guess I thought that was the way you had a party. I remember now writing invitations to my friends. But I did not tell my mother so she was the only one surprised. She was not very happy about it and I can well see why she would not have been. That was a childish thing to do.

T: To keep the record straight, how old were you then?

P: It seems as if I were nine or ten.

T: You began with relatively recent experiences and worked your way back?

P: Yes, it seems as if I skipped the whole high school period. I guess nothing important happened then. Something important did happen, though; I met Preston but we did not like each other. We had to meet again before we did.

Then I recall another instance still further back in my childhood. I remember hopping freight trains with some other children and I did not want my mother to find it out. It is perfectly logical that I didn't want my mother to know. When I recall that, I almost shudder lest Judy find out, since trains pass by our campus all the time and she might hop one. I guess Mother had warned me to stay away, but obviously I disobeyed her.

And then I go back to something that might or might not be significant, back to age eight or nine. I guess I mentioned to you that one time my folks got me a tiny puppy, thinking I would get over my fear, but I didn't want it. I was afraid of it. I remember something about my washing the front porch. There was a pail of water and my sister Wilma, six years younger than I, was playing on the porch with me and the little puppy got up on the porch. Ordinarily the little puppy would not be in the yard at the same time I was. That is how I felt about him. If I was in the front yard, he would be in the back. He got in the water, as I recall, ran out the open gate, across the street, had a fit, and died. I had mixed emotions at the time. I was sorry it had died, but glad it was gone.

The last incident I have written down goes still further back. I was a very small child. Some adult was holding me in her arms. There was a dog jumping around her feet. I had no fear of the dog.

I noted here that I was awake from 1:30 to somewhere around 4:15. It was imperative at the time that I jot these things down. I don't know if they have any connection. Something compelled me to write them down.

Sometime after that I went to sleep and I had a terrifying dream. I was sitting on a low front porch like at Mother James's about a foot from the ground, and there was a large dog with a very vicious face attacking me. He was large and muscular and threw himself at me, knocking me over and biting me. I do not know if I was an adult or a child. I am surprised that I am not saying to the dog, "Go away," but instead I am trying to quiet him, but I am terribly afraid, trembling all over. The dog got quiet, sat in my lap, and I am stroking his fur. I awoke to find myself saying out loud, "Down, down, down," in a gentle tone of voice. After that terrifying dream, I was actually trembling all over; much of the depression seemed to have left. I do not know what that means. I told my husband that I hoped it meant that I was winning the "dog fight." [7]

Then Wednesday, that was last night, I should have had a very pleasant dream since I went to the concert earlier in the evening. I dreamed something else. I slept last night, too.

I guess I am deriving some fringe benefits. I lost about eight pounds. I had thought I would have to diet.

[7] There is a question of whether this dream complies with the suggestion of the last session that she have a parallel dream to the one reported concerning her sister. The emotional tone seems to have some similarity. In this instance, identification with the mother-in-law seems to provide the patient with the support originally derived from her older sister.

T: That is certainly looking at the bright side of it. I see what you mean when you said I gave you a lot of homework.

P: I worked hard, didn't I?

T: Yes, very much so.

P: I still have a book to read too. I have to find out "why." Have you read *The Importance of Living* by Lin Yutang? I noticed when I got the book today it was copyrighted in 1937. He seems to be a modern Chinese philosopher living in New York. During class this afternoon, between helping students, I read a little of the preface. It looks pretty interesting, but I have got to find out why it was *that* interesting because I was very busy that last year of college. Preston and I were doing everything we could to get ourselves into a financial position for him to go on to school. We both worked very hard but I still found time to read that book three times.

T: It does seem to have been very important to you.

P: For some reason, yes.

T: Maybe I can help you understand its importance to you.

P: Well, I am going to read it and try to find out. I don't know what his philosophy was.

T: Do you consciously recall the homework assignment I gave you?

P: No, except that I was supposed to record dreams. Is that what you told me to do? You must have. You did, didn't you? Did you tell me something else to do?

T: Yes, and apparently you have done it. During the hour we will try to understand what your unconscious has been saying to you in these memories. Do you see any unifying theme running through them?

P: Yes, I seem to be irked with my dad for some reason but he and I got along real well. Yet, I can understand something about it. When I was home, I missed my husband terribly. It was only a couple of days after that I lost the baby. I just didn't feel well physically or mentally. The reason I wanted to go see my husband's brother was that I have always felt closer to his family than my own. I was real irked about Dad not helping. Before his death I talked to him about many things but this just didn't seem important to talk about to him or I would have told him I was sorry about the way I felt. He may not have known how I felt, but I did, and I suspect maybe that bothered me. It was nothing I brooded over, but two or three times I have kind of wished I had talked to him about it.

The incidents when my mother was displeased with me, I think she had grounds for — probably I gave her a pretty rough time.

T: You have given me a lot of material. Where would you like to begin under hypnosis?

P: I don't know. Nothing seems to be more important than anything else.

T: Well, why don't you sit back and relax?

P: I am tired enough to relax today, I really am. Nothing stands out as being important except the dream about the dog and I hope I don't have to go through that again. But of course if I have to, that is all right.

[Hypnosis is induced through the tapping method.]

T: May I say again before we get into the material today that you have been a very cooperative, industrious patient? While I think we both agree that we want to resolve this problem as quickly as possible, I do not want to overburden you by setting too fast a pace. If I overestimate your strength, feel free to let me know. I want to work at your pace as fast as you can but not too fast. Anytime I give you too much to do, feel free to tell me.

I think you must be very much aware now that this original problem, your fear of dogs, is merely a surface problem. It is like digging up a tree whose roots are deeply imbedded and go in all directions, leaving only the trunk exposed. Your fear of dogs marks the spot where these roots are buried. Last time we spent most of the hour back in your early childhood, when you were four and five years old. We uncovered a very disturbing experience: the death of your little sister for which you were blamed, an injustice in that your little dog actually caused the accident. After she died your mother continued to blame you. You also reported a second dream concerned with the death of your older sister. We did not have time to go into that. The session before that, you were confronted with another disturbing experience, the death of your babies. It seemed we had to work through one experience to get back to the earlier.

Last time I gave you the instructions that your unconscious would begin to call up and fit together the pieces of this jigsaw puzzle. It was noted that a theme of death ran through much of what we had talked about. I suggested you would recall a series of events, related in some way, which would help us to understand what had happened to you over a period of years, culminating in your present problem. The instructions meant to give us a developmental point of view. There is possibly some vital link between these memories you reported at the beginning of the hour. Let's recall those memories in turn and as we do, I want you to relax and allow yourself to freely associate to them. Don't consciously direct your thinking but instead report on the thoughts and feelings stimulated by them.

You first mentioned remembering about your child's death and then your father's death ten years later. You recalled an incident in which you were angered at the fact that he did not help you take your car from the garage. What comes to mind when you think about this memory?

P: A feeling of hopelessness.

T: You felt powerless in the situation? Now completely give over your imagination. I want you to again picture the crystal ball. Gaze intently into it, and as you do, this scene returns in all its vividness. It is in October, 1943. You are at the garage. You are having trouble getting the car out.

P: I just can't get it out. I had not been driving very long. I didn't know how to turn it right. I thought Dad would help me. I went to his store, but he could not leave.

T: How do you feel?

P: I wish he would, I felt he should have! It was his lunch hour at the store and it was closed. But he had some groceries to put up on the shelves. I resented it. He should have helped me.

T: How resentful did you feel?

P: I don't know but I was very unhappy.

T: You are in the scene itself, let yourself merge so that you are actually living it. Now it is October, 1943; you have gone to get your father. He has told you he is too busy. You are going back to the garage. Describe the feeling that dominates you.

P: I just don't like it! I am real provoked at Dad! I will just get the car out myself. I wish I had not come home. There wasn't anything else to do. We could not afford to keep our little house. I could have gone to his mother's home but my mother did not want me to.

T: This feeling of resentment toward your father — I want you to let it build up now so that you experience it as intensely as you felt then — so that you feel now as you felt then.

Memories spin before your eyes. Time is passing. In a moment it will stop and you will be in a situation where you felt the same way about your father. Now you are in another scene where you felt the same way.

P: I am just a child, not too old. I am unhappy. My dad spanked me. About the only time he ever did because Mother always disciplined us. He spanked me for leaving a light on that I could not turn off. I could not reach it.

T: Your father spanked you for something you couldn't help?

P: I could not reach the light.

T: He spanked you for something that wasn't your fault. Why did he feel so angry?

P: I don't know, but that is what he spanked me for.

T: How old are you?

P: Nine or ten.

T: When he spanked you that time you had the same feeling that you experienced at the garage?

P: Yes, I did.

T: Time is spinning by again. You are still dominated by the same feeling. When I stop time now you will be in another situation in which you felt the same way, not necessarily with your father but in the same feeling. Where are you?

P: Now it is much later. It is in my sister's kitchen after her death. Everybody was there. The funeral isn't until next week. This is Sunday; she died Saturday. The funeral is Monday or Tuesday. Everybody has gone back to St. Louis to do the things that have to be done. My husband and I stayed with my brother-in-law. It is noon time. My husband asked Gordon where he would like to eat. He preferred dinner at home. I am alone in the kitchen. I don't know her kitchen. I have been in her house only once before. I feel frustrated. I don't know how to go about preparing dinner. Some of my family should have stayed with me. There is her apron. I am so unhappy; I sit down and cry. I feel hopeless about this situation. I don't know how to go about working in her kitchen. I feel terribly hopeless about it and I feel that some of my family should have stayed with me. I wished Preston would come into the kitchen with me.

T: So the feeling here is —?

P: I am resentful.

T: You are resentful because you feel mistreated and imposed upon?

P: I guess so. At least I wish someone were there to help me. I think they all had good excuses for going back to St. Louis. No, I don't feel imposed upon. It is just a situation I wish I wasn't in. I feel helpless in a situation of this kind. If I could just ask my sister what to do.

T: This is a situation in which you need help?

P: Yes, certainly I need help. I don't know how to maneuver in her kitchen. Perhaps I do feel imposed upon. Yes, perhaps I do feel it is an imposition to ask me to prepare dinner when I feel so alone and don't know how to operate. I suspect I do feel imposed upon. It would have been simpler to eat in a restaurant or a hotel.

T: It is a situation in which you might reasonably expect the members of your family to help you, but they don't.

P: I guess so. I don't blame them for going back to St. Louis, but maybe I expect Preston or Gordon to come out to the kitchen to help me.

T: That gives us the first piece or two of our complex jigsaw. Let's take up another piece. I want you to look into the crystal ball. As I talk, each piece will appear vividly in turn, and they will begin to arrange themselves into some sort of pattern. As you look at them and see them becoming organized you will become increasingly aware of the meaning of these memories. Are you looking into the crystal ball?

P: Yes.

T: We have the first couple of pieces. Your child's death in 1943, your dad's death in 1953, and then the incident about the garage. The next is about teasing Mother James about what you would do if your husband left you. Another occurs in the summer of 1939. You are unhappy because your father objected to your spending time with another young man. You feel hurt because of your father's objections. Another piece appears — the last year of college, this book, *The Importance of Living*, you read it several times. It seemed to have some special significance to you. Graduation with honors, disappointment that no member of your family came. Now you work your way back in time, the surprise birthday party which displeases your mother. Hopping a freight train and not wanting your mother to know. Remember your folks giving you a little dog you did not want? It runs up on the front porch and then across the street, has a fit and dies. One final piece still further back, a dog jumps up while someone is holding you in her arms. Can you see the pieces there? Look at them. There is a last organization taking place. The pieces falling into place, then slowly stopping, each in its *right* position, the place where it is meant to be. Tell me now what you see.

P: It is an odd sort of things. I must see it and grasp it but it is like a concept you cannot quite express.

T: Don't try to force it just yet. Look at the pieces and absorb their meaning. Allow yourself to begin to talk about them without having to completely recognize the meaning. Talk freely.

P: Well, I feel that I would like to please my family, but I don't know how. I would like for them to approve of the things I do. And then it seems less important to please them.

T: You can absorb more of the meaning now.

P: It is like Judy when she is doing her homework. I need a hint. It seems that I almost can and then I can't. Perhaps I am feeling sorry for myself because I can't gain approval for what I do. Is that there too?

T: Somehow you didn't ever feel quite secure and accepted by the members of your family.

P: Yes, definitely that is there. It is a conscious feeling, I don't have to look for that. I found security in my husband's family. Many times I have laughed and told him I married him for his family. His mother was closer to me than my own mother. His sister and brother seem like my own sister and brother. Certainly I found security that I know I never had. I always felt very insecure. I had a very definite inferiority complex. If I didn't know it then, I did later after I looked back. Down through the years I have lost much of it and was able to feel confident about the things I wanted to do, achieve, and be.

T: So today it is no longer so necessary to please the members of your family.

P: That's right. I no longer feel that way. I am sure I felt resentful towards my mother. Looking back to my first baby's death, I can't help feeling resentful for my mother not looking out for me. It was my first pregnancy and I didn't know how careful I had to be. I worked awfully hard at Dad's store. I lifted heavy things. The doctor said that was why the baby came early. I think I resented her not telling me at the time. As I grew older I came to understand that she didn't realize how careful I had to be. She had eight children without any difficulty. But, yes, at the time I resented that.

T: You often felt intensely resentful in those days, but later apparently with greater objectivity you have been able to excuse her?

P: Oh, yes.

T: Again focus your attention on these pieces there before you. All these pieces, all of them important, all of them related. The death of your child, your father's death, the resentment at the garage, the resentment of your father telling you not to associate with this young man, the book. . . .

P: Oh, yes, the book. Yes, now I know why it is important. I will read it and find out really why, but I think it helped me to understand and not be so resentful. It didn't matter after I had read it, that my family objected to my going to college, of my plans in life. Before then I thought I should not have spent my money going to school. It was during the depression. My father lost his job. He had been a fur inspector for many years; they did not need him any longer. I thought I should not go to college; I should stay at home. When I lived there I paid board but I was putting some away for college. It was important I go to college. Preston and I were going together and were going to get married. He was to be in educational work and I wanted to be acceptable as an educator's wife. I *had* to go to college. It didn't matter after I read the book whether they cared or not. I looked at it differently.

T: This book freed you from a feeling of responsibility to your family?

P: Yes.

T: I want you to look into the crystal ball, at the book. The wind riffles the pages. In a moment the wind will stop and the book will remain open at a paragraph, a page which was important to you, one of the things which you found in the book which helped you. The pages have stopped riffling. The book lies open. Look at the page. Can you see the printing?

P: Yes.

T: Look at it carefully. Read what it says there on the page.

P: Well, it is odd that it should be in that book. It is a Shakespearean quotation.

T: Read it, please.

P: "To thine own self be true. . . . Strive to achieve your ideals." Is that really in the book?

T: Read what is on the page.

P: It surprises me. "Happiness comes by believing in one's self."

T: Do you see anything else?

P: No.

T: You are beginning to understand why this book was important to you?

P: Yes.

T: Let us go on, I want you to "see" the whole picture. Still other pieces. The surprise birthday party, hopping a freight, a tiny puppy. You are on that front porch, someone is there with you. Who is that?

P: That is Wilma. She came along after Velma's death.

T: Describe to me exactly what you are doing.

P: I have a toy broom in my hand. I am scrubbing the porch and Wilma comes up on the porch. She is quite small. She is crawling up on the porch and the puppy comes up on the porch. I am afraid of it. I don't like it. I wish they had not given it to me. I am afraid the puppy will hurt her and I wish the puppy would go away. It goes away, has a fit, and dies.

T: Tell me again. The puppy comes on the porch. What do you do?

P: I grab Wilma and tell the puppy to go away.

T: What does it do?

P: It drinks some water out of the pail. It is not a pail, it is a flat pan, and it runs out the open gate. I am afraid and I go down and close the gate. Then Mother comes upstairs from down in the basement and the man from across the street says the puppy is in their garage — no, a shed — in back and is having a fit, and it died. I was afraid they would blame me for its death, but I was glad it wasn't coming back anymore. I felt relieved it was gone.

T: How old are you?

P: I am eight.

T: Did anyone blame you?

P: I don't believe they did.

T: I want you to be eight years old again back there that day, that time. I want you to experience the same feelings and thoughts you had then. You are there on the porch with Wilma, the little puppy comes on the porch. What do you feel?

P: I am afraid he will hurt her and if he does they will blame me for it.

T: If the puppy hurts your little sister they might blame you. Where does this feeling come from?

P: I think it comes from the previous incident, the incident from last week.

T: You are afraid the puppy will hurt your little sister. Do you now know where this fear comes from at *that* time, when you are eight?

P: No, I don't.

T: Do you remember Velma?

P: Oh, yes, I remember Velma.
T: Do you remember what happened to her?
P: I remember, she died.
T: Do you remember how she died?
P: Not as an eight-year-old!
T: You are sure you do not know? As this eight-year-old you do not remember the dog knocking her down?
P: I don't think so.
T: Try to again recapture the feeling of that time, the puppy. What do you feel about that puppy?
P: I can't stand to touch it. It feels so alive. When they made me touch it I would wrap a towel around it so I did not feel it so keenly. I didn't want to touch it.
T: Didn't you know then why you had such a fear of the dog?
P: No, I just didn't like to touch it.
T: The meaning of these memories which occurred the last few days will continue to come to you now and in the next few days so you will attain an ever increasing understanding of the sequence and what it means.

You told of a terrifying dream which occurred after the recall of these memories. The meaning associated with this dream begins to make itself known to you. You begin to understand the meaning of this dream and its relationship to the memories that you had been reliving in the hours just before. Somehow, again, all this is related, all a part of a picture and the dream was a natural consequence of these memories. Tell me what comes to mind.
P: I don't know. A sort of feeling that in any struggle . . . maybe I can explain it more graphically. It is like being in a tunnel in a train. Sort of like a thing accomplished. I can't quite express what I feel. Like someone on a train and it is about to come out on the daylight side.
T: The dream represents a feeling of accomplishment?
P: I think the dream depicts a struggle that has been going on in myself, my fear of dogs. I think we are about to overcome that fear. I hope that is what it means. Even though it was terrifying, I kept the dog from attacking me.
T: You may wonder if this was a memory of a real experience. I want you to relax and see if there were any memories where you were actually, physically attacked by a dog. If there are, that memory will now come to mind. If not, I think it is safe to assume you are depicting an inner conflict. I am going to count gradually

to ten; if such a memory exists, you will remember before I reach ten. One . . . two . . . three. . . .

P: I see a situation. It is one I had forgotten but it is not actually as violent as that. It was in the summer during my college years. I was working at St. Louis for Lever Brothers. They had girls going from door to door giving a bar of Lux soap and Lux flakes. We were not to go in a yard with a vicious dog. I got in this yard with a fence and gate around it. A dog came running around the side of the house. I got to the porch door, between the screen and the door, I saw the dog coming, but I was in no danger. I was afraid but not too afraid because I had the screen door before me. The lady of the house came to the door and put the dog into the back yard. This wasn't too frightening an experience.

T: I am going to continue the count. If you have any memories where you were actually attacked, they will come to mind. [Counts to ten.]

P: [With a note of finality] There are none.

T: I think we can be fairly confident, then, that this dream is symbolic rather than factual. I think our time is about up for today. Is there anything additional you would like to bring up before we terminate?

P: Not about this, but I am going to the dentist on Tuesday. Why don't you make me not so conscious of the vibrations because I am very sensitive to them? Not the pain but the vibrations. When Dr. Segerson fills a tooth he knows I am very conscious of the vibrations. Let's see if you can do something about it.

T: It might be interesting to try. You would really like to do it very much?

P: I would like to try.

T: You say you are not afraid of the pain but you dislike the vibrations?

P: I don't like pain, but I am not afraid of it. When we have a bad filling to do he uses novocaine but he cannot eliminate the vibration. I think that is why I dislike the dentist so much. It is sort of like loud music.

T: I think you can take yourself deep enough to make the suggestions effective.

The patient was given the suggestion to take herself very deeply. Suggestions were given that when she sat in the dentist's chair and he put the drill in her mouth, she would find herself completely preoccupied with the crystal ball and in it she would observe a series of very pleasant scenes. No noise or pain, regardless of its intensity, would divert her attention. At the same time she was instructed that she would give every appearance of being wide awake and that she would be able to completely cooperate with the dentist in his procedures. The subject was also given the suggestion that she be amnesic to instructions given for the dentist.

Before the patient was awakened she was given additional suggestions to the effect that the pieces of her life relating to her problem would continue to fall in place, so that she would have an increasing conscious and unconscious awareness of the pattern of her life. At the same time she was cautioned to proceed at a more moderate pace. The last suggestion given was that another session or two should complete this treatment series. The patient was then awakened.

T: Was that a restful sleep?

P: Oh, yes.

T: [Humorously] It was the least I could do after having caused you so many sleepless nights lately.

P: It is a small price to pay for all I am getting out of this, especially the eight pounds I've lost. I am afraid that all the girls will want to come here for treatment when they find out how I lost it. Several of them have said to me, "Why, Mrs. James, have you been dieting?" I talked to them before about several reducing diets and they probably think I have been testing them out.

T: Did you tell anyone about your coming here for treatment?

P: Just my husband. He told me he had talked to the president of the college and the business manager and they were very much interested. I sat by the president last night at the concert. I am glad I wasn't sitting by him last week when I had such a difficult time keeping awake.

T: You didn't find you were bothered by tapping noises this week?

P: Oh, my, no. I got through the classes without any difficulty. If I come through this satisfactorily I see no reason why people should not know. People think that an emotional problem is something to be ashamed of rather than to understand. I knew I always had a problem, something I could not get through myself. My husband said that following the last session he thought I had uncovered the source of my difficulty. I told my husband in the beginning that you might want to commit me and if you did, it was all right because they have a potter's wheel in O.T. and I don't have access to one.

You know, I don't know whether I am being objective or subjective anymore. Until all this began I had myself diagnosed as a very happy, optimistic individual, but I am just not sure now that I am. I expect I will emerge as what I thought I was. I can see in the things I went back to dig up, especially the letters in the trunk, that I had some pretty troubled times.

T: You mentioned thinking of yourself as a very happy and well-adjusted person. I see no reason for you to change this opinion of yourself. Freud once said that people are normal because of the success of their repression. They are able to lock away a great many of the painful experiences which the neurotic fails to do. I would certainly assume that you were normal and as such had successfully locked away those things that bothered you.

P: In college I was trying very hard to find myself. I took every psychology and philosophy course they had. My husband was kidding me the other night. He said he thought it was because the philosophy professors always gave me A's, but I think I was trying to find myself. I had to find out why I had this fear.

T: Rather than looking at this present experience as any indication that you are not a normal person, I think the positive and realistic way to look at it is that you have the rare opportunity here to do a lot of tidying up. Nobody completely plans their lives. In a sense they just grow up and a lot of messy things happen which you sweep under the rug or hide in the closet. Here you can open the closet door and put these things in order.

P: I really do feel that way about it.

Session VI, February 10

The patient looked more relaxed than she had in the past week and she asked if she should have done some written homework since she had not. Memories continued to come back to her but at a reduced rate and intensity so that she was generally more comfortable. She brought in a pencil sketch of her daughter

Judy, drawn on February 4, which she thought reflected her feelings of depression at the time. She stated that when shown to friends one of them had remarked, "What happened to Judy? I have never seen her look so sad." She also brought in two old photographs. The first was taken with Velma, and in this she looked happy and animated. The second was taken with Wilma and in this she appeared rather pinched and unhappy. She commented that this feeling characterized her memory of her early childhood.

She also reported in detail on her experience with the dentist that morning. In going to his office she debated whether or not to allow him to use novocaine. She found he had the needle already prepared. One rather large hidden cavity had been discovered by X-ray. However, she decided against using novocaine and somewhat to her surprise and very much to the surprise of Dr. Segerson, she evidenced and felt no pain throughout the entire proceedings. She had no difficulty seeing and concentrating on the crystal ball. (She called it the "magic ball.") She felt somewhat annoyed when Dr. Segerson insisted on talking and distracting her attention. Nevertheless, the suggestions were completely effective. Apparently his curiosity was aroused by the whole procedure but in spite of the fact that he tried to draw her out, she did not reveal to him how she had accomplished this control of pain. He asked if she had been practicing Yoga. Her reaction to this was that he might categorize hypnosis in the same manner and she would not tell him, although she might at some later time. She was quite impressed with the possibilities in the use of hypnosis for the control of pain.

She brought with her a copy of Lin Yutang's *Importance of Living*, and she was asked whether she had read and now understood the importance of this book to her during her college days.

P: I was going to a religious school at the time I read this book. They taught me that you had to be perfect and if you weren't God was out there and would punish you. I couldn't accept that. I remember now that I look back on it, that many of the young ministerial students who are now prominent ministers were kind of concerned because I didn't follow right down the line. I just couldn't accept it! I think this book sort of gave me the philosophy of life that I needed and philosophy of religion too, for that matter.

After reading the book again, I was surprised to find that Lin Yutang is really a pagan and I am far from being a pagan, but then a Chinese pagan is not too far from a liberal Christian. My family was Protestant and I grew up in a Catholic neighborhood, and many of my best friends were Catholic. So I just could not accept that unless you were this or that denomination you did not get to heaven. My very best friend in high school and her mother and family were Lutheran so there again was a barrier, and all during high school I had worked for a Jewish family so I just didn't have the right associations to make me accept the indoctrination that the college gave me. But this book gave me what I needed, and I think I followed along with it pretty much. Would you like to hear part of it, just a little bit that I marked here that seemed most pertinent?

In this section, "Why I Am a Pagan," he says: "Religion is always an individual, personal thing. Every person must work out his own views on religion. If he is sincere, then God will not blame him however it turns out. Every man's religious experience is valid for himself. For as I have said, it is not something to be argued about. This is a story about a Llama's soul struggling with its problems as told in a sincere manner and as such will always be of benefit to other people. That is why speaking about religion I must get away from generalities in telling my personal story."

Then he tells why he became a pagan. He had been in a very religious family. His father was a pastor but he could not accept the — well — sort of things I could not accept, that if you pray and ask God for something that he might disregard the needs of maybe a whole town to give you a miracle. That sort of thing was in his thinking too. He goes on to say, "As a condition of belief concerning life in the universe, that in which I feel natural and at ease without having to be at war with myself. In Taoistic phraseology it is but being intellectually sincere with oneself in the universe according to one's light, and I believe no one can be natural and happy unless he is sincere with himself." Then he says, "A Chinese pagan is one who starts out with his earthly life as all he can or need bother about. This is to live as intently and happily as long as his life lasts, often has a sense of the poignant sadness of life and faces it clearly, has a keen appreciation of the beautiful and the good of human life wherever we find them, and regards doing good as its own satisfactory reward. I admit, however, that he feels a slight pity and contempt for the religious man who does good in order to get to heaven and who, by implication, would not do good if he weren't lured by heaven or threatened by hell. If this statement is correct, I believe there are a great many pagans in this country, more than they themselves are aware of. The modern liberal Christian and the pagan are very close, differing only when they start talking about God. As I look at it at present the differences in spiritual life between a Christian and a pagan are simply this, the Christian believer lives in a world governed and watched over by God to whom he has a constant personal relationship and, therefore, in a world presided over by a kindly Father." And he goes on to say that "Peace of mind is that mental condition in which you have accepted the worst."

I think that is what was in that book for me. Down through my life probably after this, I sort of felt like, and I have often told students that, to me it is not *what* happened to you but *how* you reacted to what happened to you in life. I don't know if that is very valid, but to me it is.

T: How can you summarize, then, the influence this book had on you during your college days?

P: I think it was just this turmoil within myself of trying to not be too different from the bulk of these ministerial students and of finding my own self religiously. Perhaps that was it. I don't know, I can't think of any other reason.

T: This book gave you the support necessary to find your own answer to these problems?

P: I think so. Does that make sense?

T: Certainly.

P: Well, to me it did.

T: Last time you also related this book to the help it had given you in regaining your independence from the opinions of your family.

P: Yes, I think that struggle definitely went on. I grew up always wanting to please, at least not displease my family. In anything I did I wanted their approval. I just could not do things without feeling it was all right with them. I can remember being amused at my younger sister. She didn't give a care about what the folks thought. I remember one time especially she and the man she is now married to and another couple went on a weekend trip to Detroit and

my mother and father were so against it. I think the other couple
was married. I couldn't see how she could do it. I think this book
gave me a freedom from a lot of things.

T: Freedom to be yourself?

P: That's right.

T: Incidentally, did you run across the quotation from Shakespeare?

P: I haven't yet. I have a few more pages to go of it, if it is in here.

T: I wonder if that quotation from Shakespeare isn't there in essence.

P: Yes, I wondered that when I read it.

T: You should not expect every detail of every memory to be absolutely correct. I think the memories we've recovered are probably
correct in the sense that they convey the feeling experienced.

P: That is the way I felt about it. The Shakespearean quotation may
not be in here but it, too, was probably important to me.

T: How about the problem we worked on so hard last time, putting
the pieces of this jigsaw together? How these memories were related and in turn relate to your earliest experiences? Do you think
you have a better understanding today?

P: I am not sure. Do I have to remember everything of my life that
ever happened to me? I was amused at my husband at noon. I told
him I seemed to remember *everything*. He asked me then if I remembered a certain green dress I wore when we were engaged
and which he liked very much. I had completely forgotten it but
that started a whole train of thought about other dresses so I told
him not to remind me of anything else, please. It seemed like I was
remembering and remembering and remembering.

As one grows older I think the years sort of run together but they
are all straightened out now, things which have been long forgotten, interesting instances and some not so interesting.

T: Do you have a feeling that you would like to stop this remembering process?

P: Well, not if it is necessary to get to the bottom of this thing because that to me is most important. Incidentally, why was I free of
that fear for just a few minutes? The fear of the dog that morning
and then it came back.

T: Well, let's put it this way, it is a sign of progress that you were
free if just for a few minutes. You have had this fear for a whole
lifetime. There are so many associations reinforcing it that it isn't
realistic to expect to get rid of it immediately.

P: I guess I had hoped I would.

T: What you should find is that as you face and understand these disturbing memories, you will be more comfortable and will have

more control over your fear. This will depend on how completely you face these past experiences.

P: I would like to work hard and get rid of the fear entirely.

T: I have this feeling about it. The first few sessions we covered considerable ground in a short period of time. If we had attacked this problem the conventional way we might be months away from the recovery of these same memories. You have found going back and reliving was more painful than anticipated, and as a result I purposely slowed down the pace so you would have a little more rest.

P: I think I needed it. I was just worn out Saturday. I rested all day. I didn't know whether it was working so hard on this or the big party I had Friday night. It is a good thing you slowed down on this because I could not slow down on the party. Although my mind kept working on these memories, there seemed to be no compulsion to write them down as I had previously felt.

T: Is it possible that you are working a little too hard?

P: No, I don't think so. I usually attack a problem pretty vigorously. If I have something to do, I usually want to get it done.

T: As you have shown in these sessions. Are you aware of any continuing change in your feelings about dogs?

P: I don't know why but I think that I have been helped. The fear is still there, perhaps not as acutely.

T: Frankly, I would have been surprised if it wasn't. Have you had the courage to try an experiment with dogs again?

P: I haven't had the opportunity. The only dog that has been near today was the dog on the corner, a real vicious dog that is ordinarily kept tied. It came near my husband and me. I don't think he felt much more comfortable than I. I haven't had a chance to meet a dog that was, I started to say that was human, I didn't mean to say that, that wasn't vicious.

T: It is realistic to be afraid of big, vicious dogs but you have been particularly afraid of small, active, friendly ones too. You might try testing yourself again.

P: Yes, because I want to get rid of that fear.

Hypnosis was induced by tapping method at this juncture. The memory of her little sister's death was recalled to her. It was suggested that she would become increasingly aware of the influence of this early experience. It was next suggested that she might momentarily explore what it was specifically about the movie, *The Three Faces of Eve*, that had prompted her to finally seek professional assistance. The situation in which she had viewed the movie was reinstated by suggestion. She was told to look at the movie theater screen and upon a given signal she would view selected scenes which had the deepest personal meaning to her. The first scene she recalled was of the young woman in the doctor's office.

P: He was talking to her. The husband was outside not understanding her at all. She seems to be saying "I can't help myself." He is asking her if she realizes the things she did, about the various escapades and hurting the child. She says she doesn't remember and couldn't help herself.

[Three other scenes are then recalled in rapid succession.]

P: She is in a rooming house trying to find herself. She will not go to her husband until she does. She feels he is not very understanding. . . . Now she is playing in the yard with a little girl. Just playing ball. . . . The scene in the car with the child and her husband and having freedom and security. It is on the way home after treatment is over.

T: [These four scenes are then reinstated through suggestion.] As you look at this first scene there on the screen it will begin to change. The figures will melt away and be replaced by other people. That is *you* there in the scene. It will become you and your own situation, the situation in your own life that was directly related to the one on the screen. What do you see now? Can you see yourself?

P: Yes.

T: Who is there with you?

P: A doctor. I guess you, yes, it is you.

T: What is going on? What is being said?

P: It is like our first meeting here when you didn't know whether you could help me and I hoped that you could.

T: Now the second scene. The woman is alone in the rooming house, determined not to go back to her husband until the problem is straightened out. Watch the figures melt away to be replaced by a situation of significance to you.

P: I think it is all those years when I felt misunderstood by my mother and I wanted to tell her things which I should have told her. There were instances when I might have been in danger but I could never approach my mother. She never understood. I could never talk to her about things that mattered.

T: The scene depicts your feelings of being misunderstood, not being able to get through to people, particularly your mother? Let's go on to the next scene now.

P: I see the scene where she is hurting her child.

T: Now it is changing. It is you. What situation are you in?

P: I am talking to Judy. She wants a puppy dog very badly. She tells me she is lonesome. She has no brother or sister. I don't want her to be lonely. I don't want to hurt her by being lonely.

T: You don't want her to go through what you did. Now the scene in the yard where the mother and child are playing ball. Tell me about it.

P: It is just the mother and the child happily playing together.

T: As you would like to play with Judy.

The movie scene depicting the patient's early childhood experience in which the grandmother had died was reinstated. The patient recalled it vividly. Contrary to the therapist's anticipation, this scene seemed to have no deep personal significance for her. She did experience "a feeling of kinship to the child that the parents did not understand."

T: What was the paramount feeling that this movie left you with?

P: A feeling of hope that I could be helped with my problem.

T: And at the time what was your understanding of the problem that confronted you?

P: For many years I have had the feeling that if I could talk to someone that knew how to dig up the past, I would not be afraid of dogs anymore.

T: Did you perceive your problem as specifically that of a fear of dogs or was it broader?

P: No, a fear of dogs.

T: All of your problems were, in a sense, wrapped up in your fear of dogs?

P: Yes, I think that as an adolescent I was afraid of people. Undoubtedly, I had a terrific inferiority complex. I did not care to mix. But in my college years that started on the wane, and after I was married this helped me overcome much of it. If I have any inferiority complex now it is very slight. I am quite sure that as a child I had a terrific inferiority complex and a feeling of being misunderstood. My grade school teachers had long sessions with me, talking with me about various things. I guess that they saw I was a lonely child and they encouraged me to go to high school which I would never have done if they had not. In high school I lost some of it, but I still had a great deal of it. I preferred to be by myself and to draw or paint or read rather than being with most people.

T: Do you see any relationship between this pattern of behavior and this disturbing memory you have uncovered?

P: Yes, I think so, very definitely so.

T: What can you trace back to this early experience?

P: Mainly that I felt misunderstood and thought I would be misunderstood in anything else I did. So I did not want to do anything that might be misunderstood. I could not mix well with people. I felt my actions would not be understood. As I got older and became less inhibited it did not matter.

T: It took a long time before you felt strong enough to live your own life.

P: It took a long, long time and many unhappy situations because of that personality trait.

T: Do you have a better understanding of any other characteristics about yourself?

P: I am quite sure that never being close to any members of my family, particularly my mother and even my father and brothers, was another result. I think as I became a little more mature, I did not resent my parents and their reactions towards me as I had as a child and an adolescent. Later I felt sorry for them and wondered what was in my mother's life that made her so unhappy, bitter, and domineering. I asked my Aunt Ethel about her, if Mother had always been like that or only since a certain period of her life. She said no, she thought it was a trait that had been there many, many years. I felt sorry for my mother and I did not resent her anymore. I certainly don't now.

T: You have grown up enough now so that you can forgive your mother.

P: Yes, I am sure I had grown up to that stage a long time ago. I think that these sessions have also made me realize why it has always been so hard for me to discipline Judy. I know my husband has been irked many times because I could not bring myself to discipline her. I think I was always afraid I would discipline her unfairly.

I am sure I did not retain any ill feelings toward Mother or I would have noticed she resented Judy when she was living with us. I knew there was a strange relationship there between the two. I thought it was because Mother was old and an invalid and Judy was young and extremely active. I thought it was just age and childhood causing the problem, but it may have been that unconsciously she transferred her resentment from me, if she had any, if she thought I caused my sister's death, to Judy. It was pointed out to me afterward and then my brother emphasized it more by telling me that he thought Dad and Mother had resented our adopting Judy. They thought we should have taken care of them instead of adopting Judy. And then I remember unkind remarks. On one occasion she was talking about somebody's children taking care of them. She said about Judy, "Well, after all she is only an adopted child." I remember that my husband and I looked at each other and realized that Mother spoke a little less of an adopted child.

T: In the last few weeks you have apparently done a lot of thinking about the pattern of your life.

P: Yes, I really have.

T: You see more clearly how you grew and developed.

P: I think so but I think I had thought a lot about it even before, not as deeply, but I think I had thought a lot about it.

T: Meaning it had been a problem to you for some time?

P: Yes, and I felt as I grew older and studied the problems of childhood and the troubles teachers have with children that I could understand the problem child because I am pretty sure that I was one. And I suspect unconsciously I was fighting back because of this resentment that I had, the feeling of being misunderstood.

T: Let us turn our attention again to this specific fear of dogs. Last time you had a memory, apparently when you were eight, of being with your little sister Wilma, and of a puppy running on the porch. You seemed to clearly remember that you were frightened that the dog might harm your sister, but had no conscious recollection of the earlier causative experience. Let us trace back still further. Allow yourself to go very deeply asleep now. Deeper, very deep. We have talked about your memory of dogs when you were eight and also four. Someplace in between, your awareness of this earlier experience was buried. I want you to go back in time. First, I want you to recall the scene with Wilma on the back porch. Do you see it clearly?

P: Yes, I am scrubbing the porch. I have a toy broom. I am dipping it into the water. The neighbor comments I am quite Mother's little helper. My little sister is crawling up the steps. There were seven or eight steps. The dog comes. It looks like a white dog with black spots. He comes towards us. I grab my sister's hand and pull her toward me. I call to my mother because I am afraid of dogs. He takes a drink and runs into the yard across the street, not directly across but the house just to the left of the one across the street. I can see the man, I can't recall his name. His son's name was Walter. He comes back and tells my mother and me that the dog has had a fit in his shed in back and died. I feel sort of sorry and sort of glad. More glad than sorry.

T: How did you feel there on the porch when the dog came up? I want you to let yourself experience that same feeling again. You are there on the porch scrubbing with the little broom. Your sister is there and the dog comes.

P: I am afraid. I am afraid he will jump on Wilma.

T: Why are you afraid of his jumping? Tell me as you felt then.

P: I don't know. I can't distinguish between the feeling now and then.

T: Do you think you had any memory whatsoever of the earlier experience with Velma?

P: I don't think so.

T: Now relax. Go further back in time, a year or two, you are six or seven, to another situation in which there was a dog. The memory will push its way up. You are younger by a year or two. Let the picture develop, let it come: an actual memory in which you are closely associated with a dog.

P: My Aunt Nola's dog. I liked to visit my Aunt Nola, but I was afraid to go because of her dog. It was sort of jumpy.

T: You already dislike frisky dogs. What did the dog look like?

P: It wasn't very big. I don't know if it was a little bulldog or not.

T: But it was frisky.

P: Yes, jumpy. It was dark too.

T: Now can you remember a specific scene in which you were closely related with this dog?

P: [After pause] I can't.

T: I want you now to try and recapture a memory of your association with a dog at the age of five.

P: I'm at my grandfather's farm. It seems as if it is the front porch. There are lots of us there. They are urging me to touch the dog. I wish they wouldn't do that! I don't want to touch it! I wish they wouldn't do that! They say it won't hurt me.

T: Who is there with you?

P: My whole family, my grandfather, grandmother, Aunt Ethel and

Uncle Bob, my two brothers, my two cousins, no, my three cousins, and my big sister, my dad, mother, and I. I wish they wouldn't do that, it embarrasses me. I am afraid! I don't want to touch it! I don't think they should make me try it!

T: What is it doing?

P: It is jumping all around. It is a very active dog.

T: What color is it?

P: It seems dark. I am not sure but it seems there may be more than one dog.

T: What is your feeling about these dogs?

P: I am *so* afraid of them!

T: What are you afraid they will do?

P: I don't know. I am afraid they will jump on me!

T: If they jump on you, what might happen?

P: I don't know. I just don't want to touch them and I don't want them to touch me.

T: How old are you?

P: I am five.

T: You are five years old. Tell me what you remember about your little sister Velma.

P: I miss her.

T: What happened to her?

P: She died.

T: What does it mean to die?

P: To go away and not be there anymore.

T: Where do you go when you die?

P: I am not quite sure. Someplace far away.

T: Why did your sister die?

P: She fell down on a splinter.

T: Do you remember that? How do you know that?

P: I don't know. I don't know if I remembered it then or now. I don't know.

T: Let's go back further to the time when you were four, back to that tragic time. Your sister has been dead just a few days. You are very lonely, of course, and Rover, I guess he is still there?

P: I don't think he is there anymore.

T: He isn't there? What happened to him?

P: I think they gave him away.

T: Where did they take him?

P: I think to Grandpa's.

T: Do you know they took him to Grandpa's?

P: I am not real sure but I think they did.

T: How do you feel about his being gone?

P: I feel kind of guilty. My brothers wanted him there but I didn't. I just didn't want him around.

T: Why didn't you want him there anymore?

P: Because he knocked my sister down and I don't want him around anymore.

T: You were glad he was gone but felt a little guilty about it?

P: I think so. The rest of the family wanted him there. I don't think he is there anymore.

T: You are just a little girl.

P: Yes, about four or four and a half.

T: You are just a tiny girl. It must be difficult to remember. Your sister is dead. You are a lonely little girl and your mother seems to blame you for what happened. She doesn't understand or believe your story and the dog is gone now too. I want you to recapture the way you felt then, the way you feel as a little girl.

The specific memory of Rover pushing your little sister down: tell me how you think or remember this as a little girl. Tell me what happened to the memory, how long you have kept it, and then what happened to it. What did your mind do with it?

P: I feel very much alone and I feel blamed and I don't like anybody in particular. I just wish I had my little sister back and everything would be the way it was. I think maybe there is something tied up about my sister feeling so very still when I picked her up. She didn't hug me anymore. She was so still and the dog was jumping. I cannot explain it. I don't want to touch the dog anymore. I want it to go away.

T: Don't try to explain it, talk about your feelings. Your sister is so still, the dog is so full of life. How do little girls think? What did this mean to you as a little, tiny girl? Your sister is so still and the dog so frisky. What does a little girl think about those two things? It has some special meaning?

P: That her little sister can't play with her anymore. Cannot run and play and have fun. And it's the dog's fault.

T: In contrast, how about the dog?

P: He can run and play but I don't want to play with him anymore.

T: What is the feeling about your sister being so still and the dog so frisky?

P: It is not right. Something is wrong.

T: The dog took away your sister's life, her friskiness?

P: I guess that's why I don't like him.

T: His friskiness reminds you in contrast of your sister's stillness?

P: I don't know. I wonder.

T: Don't try to reason it out. Let your feelings tell you these things.

P: I don't like to touch him anymore. It makes me think of my sister. And how she doesn't move.

T: He moves so very much, your sister doesn't move at all.

P: That's it!

T: So in contrast you are always reminded of your sister's stillness?

P: I think so.

T: Can you tell me what happens to the memory of your sister and the dog pushing your little sister over, day by day? The funeral is over, you are lonely, Rover is gone. What happens to that memory?

P: It just goes away. It seems to be going away. That is the way I feel.

T: Do you remember how long it was approximately after the death of your sister that Rover was sent away?

P: I think it was soon.

T: Days or weeks?

P: I think days.

T: It is very difficult to remember so long ago. I want you to relax and go very deeply asleep. We are going to do something next which requires a very deep level, deeper than you have ever gone before. Do you understand?

P: Yes.

T: In order to accomplish this you must allow yourself to go deeper than ever before. What step would you say you are at now?

P: Thirty-five comes to mind.

T: Now we are going to count down 10 more steps. With each step you will go deeper. [The count is made.] In a moment I will awaken you. After I awaken you I want you to gaze over in the corner there. You will see a little puppy, a little *black* dog. You will see him very distinctly. He will be a very friendly little puppy. He will be interested in you and you will be interested in him. It will be as clear and vivid as the crystal ball you saw in the dentist's office. Perhaps you will recognize him, I don't know whether you will. Don't try to remember this suggestion after you awaken. [Patient is then awakened.] Did you go very deeply?

P: I must have been very deeply asleep. One doesn't snore, does one?

T: [Humorously] I wake them up when they do. How do you feel about things now?

P: I just wish I could make faster progress.

T: I feel you have done very well in this short time.

P: I am just an eager beaver. I always want to get anything I undertake done. [Patient stares intently into a corner of the office. Long pause.]

T: What are you looking at?

P: Have you got a crystal ball over there?

T: Why do you ask? What do you see?

P: Well, have you? It seems all wrapped up with that same dog.

T: Which dog is that?

P: My dog.

T: Rover? What's he doing?

P: Just sitting there, and I hope he stays there. I know he isn't there and yet I see him.

T: You know he isn't there?

P: I know it's impossible.

T: He doesn't look quite real to you?

P: Well, sort of.

T: What's he doing?

P: Just sitting there looking at me.

T: How does he look?

P: [Laughs.] He looks like I have done him an injustice, I think.

T: You want him to stay over there. You don't think you can make up with him after all these years?

P: I am not sure.

T: Do you think you can make any gesture of friendship to him?

P: I can feel sorry for him, isn't that a gesture of friendship?

T: Why don't you call him over?

P: He might come running and I wouldn't like that.

T: Why not try and see? Do you have enough courage?

P: I think I have enough courage.

T: Enough to make friends with him?

P: If he really were there, I think I could.

T: You see him, don't you?

P: But in my mind's eye only. But I really think I could if he were there.

T: You say only in your mind's eye. How real does he appear?

P: He looks very real. Like the memory this morning looked.

T: Try calling him over to you.

P: But he isn't there.

T: Why don't you try?

P: Rover, come over, come over slowly. In my mind's eye he is walking over slowly.

T: What's this about the "mind's eye"? Isn't he out there?

P: But he isn't really.

T: You don't want him to be?

P: No, I kind of think I do. I think I wish he were there.

T: Why not let him be there?

P: Yes, I think he is there. I think I would like him to come over. All right, Rover, come on over. He does.

T: Where is he?

P: He is on my lap and I am not afraid.

T: Can you stroke and pet him?

P: Yes.

T: Let me see you.

P: [Stroking.] I am not afraid. I wish he were actually there.

T: You still won't let yourself believe he is there.

P: I wish he were actually there so I could touch him. I think I would not have that repulsion of touching him with my hand.

T: Won't you let yourself feel him sitting there in your lap? This morning, if you remember, you went to the dentist. Certainly there was real physical pain. You were able to control that. Is it so much more impossible to have a little dog here with you?

P: No, I guess not really.

T: Not if you *really* want him. Where is Rover?

P: He is still in my lap. He is lying on my lap.

T: Is he friendly?

P: Yes, he feels sort of quivery underneath but I don't mind it.

T: Would you like to take him home?

P: Judy would like it and yes, I think I would.

T: You don't have to if you don't want to.

P: What would you do with a dog in your office?

T: That's a good point. [Patient and therapist laugh.]

P: Maybe you have another patient that could use him.

T: Are you sure you want him?

P: [With increasing resolution] Yes, I think I will take him home. I think so!

T: I think if you do that under the circumstances it would be a good idea to keep this between you and me.

P: [Laughs.] I think so. In my memory I can see that dog as plainly as I could see those incidents in my life this morning.

T: How real is that?

P: I think very real.

T: Why don't you take the dog along with you? We will keep it a secret between us for obvious reasons. Other people would not be able to see this dog anyway. You will find in the next day or two, until we meet again, at odd moments, especially at night, he will be there with you and you will be able to make friends with him if you want to.

P: It is sort of like Harvey's rabbit, isn't it?

T: You can say that Harvey's rabbit was a figment of his imagination but he was very real to Harvey.

P: Uh-huh.

T: If you will go back to sleep I will tell you these suggestions again. [Patient returns to sleep.] I am going to give you this little dog Rover to take with you, this little black dog of your girlhood days. You can keep him, for the next couple of days. When you come back next time, bring him with you. Only you and I will know you have this dog and how real he is to you. By yourself, especially at night alone, the little dog will be there. He will *not* make a nuisance of himself during the day by popping up at the wrong time; he has become well-trained during the years. But little Rover will be there when you want him and when you are ready to make friends with him. In this way, you can go back into the past to set right the things that went wrong, to make up with this little dog that, under the circumstances, you could not help but blame. This is a chance to become acquainted with the real Rover, not as you saw and thought about him as a little girl, but how he really was. So this will be your little dog, the same dog you had as a little girl. In the next few days, if you can let yourself, I want you to become very well acquainted with him so that you can see Rover as he really was, rather than as the way you saw him as a little girl and the way you remembered him. This will really be Rover, friendly little Rover. If you sincerely want to make friends with him, you will be able to. We both know he is only a memory but certainly your feelings about him have been very real. He will be as real as your feelings about him. Remember you will have complete control over him. He will not bother you at inconvenient times. When it is convenient for you, you will be able to renew your acquaintance with him.[8]

[8] The method employed here is an extension of the technique of hypnotically induced fantasy conflicts developed by Erickson (1935). The rationale underlying this approach is the psychoanalytic assumption that symbols have a disguise

I think you should also begin to prepare yourself for termination of these sessions. If it is acceptable to you, we will make the next session the last one for a while. You should not expect to be cured overnight but I think you will gradually lose your fear of dogs, especially if you make friends with little Rover. You will also continue to integrate and organize the pieces of your "jigsaw puzzle." By next session I want you to arrive at a decision of whether this would be a convenient place to stop for the time being. [Patient is awakened.]

P: My husband is getting real curious about the tape but I think it is better that he wait until we are finished, don't you? He isn't impatient, just curious. There must be an awful lot of tape to listen to. I want to listen to it with him, may I?

T: Certainly; I think that where hypnosis is employed the patient should have the opportunity to listen to the sessions afterward.

Session VII, February 13

P: You know back when we found this incident in my life you wondered if there was anyone I could talk to. I mentioned my mother doesn't write to me, probably because she isn't able. So I wrote some questions out, sort of in the form of an exam that she could answer yes or no. My husband told me she probably wouldn't reply. She did write, however. The only thing she confirms positively is that there was a little black dog; either she doesn't remember or, if she does, she wouldn't tell me. I think if she told me there wasn't a little black dog I would have doubted it all, because I certainly have not remembered it all these years.

T: What questions did you ask her?

P: Questions which possibly might have awakened memories she wouldn't have wanted to remember. Maybe I should not have. She remembers the dog as being called Twister but she may have forgotten.

T: [Glances at the questionnaire.] She says here that you were afraid

---

function and that conflicts are often expressed in symbolic form (dreams and neurotic symptom formation) long before they are accepted into consciousness. Erickson recognized the inability of his patient to accept a direct interpretation of his problem and, therefore, formulated it in a parallel symbolic fantasy which, while disguised to the waking mind, was apparently understood and reacted to on an unconscious level. In this manner the ego was desensitized and there was an automatic resolution of the real life problem. (Refer also to Erickson, 1944; and McDowell, 1948.)

of dogs all of your life.

P: She has stubbornly maintained I am afraid of dogs because of pre-natal markings. I don't believe it and never have. I don't think she would admit otherwise. Mother is not one to admit she is wrong. The interesting thing is, if I was afraid of dogs all my life, why were there dogs in the family until I was four years old? I can remember them talking about many dogs before then but there were never any dogs after that except the one they got me which I didn't want. So I don't know. But the little black dog being there, she remembered that.

T: You say you might doubt the whole experience?

P: Well, you wonder, can your mind make up things? Surely my mind didn't make up an awful tale like this, did it?

T: Not unless there was some purpose that isn't apparent.

P: Why would it?

T: What purpose would you have in horrifying yourself in the way you have?

P: Yes, it wasn't a regular dream. I shuddered about it everytime I thought about it! Most dreams you forget when you wake up but I didn't forget that one. It was so vivid I would cringe each time I thought about it.

T: Your feelings tell you that something like this must have occurred, regardless of whether we have it correct in all detail. The intense emotions accompanying this dream probably testify to its validity better than anything else.

P: And there was another thing. I remember that sometime in my life another incident took place that Mother denies. We were all lined up and walking to a door and when I got to the door, something knocked, I don't know what. I have asked my mother about that in the past and she has always insisted there was no such incident. But I know there was, I can remember *it*, but I didn't know what it was connected with. So I don't know [about the questionnaire]. It could be she has forgotten. It's been many years and many things have happened to her.

T: Or it could be that unpleasant as the situation was, she hasn't wanted to face it.

P: Yes, I thought of that too. It could well be. But to me the fact that she remembered the little black dog was something. The little dog I saw wasn't red or tan or brown but black! Incidentally, my husband thinks I have been helped a great deal. Night before last we had a ham bone and he said if I would wrap it, he would carry it out to the incinerator, and without thinking I said, "Let's keep it and we will give it to some dog." So he thinks I have improved a great deal. I don't ever remember thinking before I would save a bone for a dog.

Something else is interesting. It was so hard for me to discipline Judy. Yet I would read all those books that children must be disciplined and I knew that they must, but every time I had to I would stay awake nights and think, am I doing right? The other day she really gave me trouble and I disciplined her without a twinge of conscience. I think before that I was afraid I would discipline her unjustly because I had been.

T: You were identifying with her, remembering how you felt?

P: I guess so but she isn't going to like you now because I can spank her and I couldn't used to. I know my husband used to be irked with me because it was so hard for me to discipline her. But it isn't hard now. When she needs it I know I am not treating her unjustly, that I am doing something that she needed.

Maybe I can be a normal human being now and not have all those frustrations and fears. In looking back, I know I had a terrific inferiority complex. But my husband knew just how to deal with me, I guess.

T: He has helped you a lot. Undoubtedly you have grown considerably these last few years. I think you can look upon this experience as another step in your growth.

P: I hope so. Of course, the happy day will be when I can be on friendly terms with all the puppy dogs.

T: Tell me how you and Rover got along.

P: Oh, just fine. There was a slightly strained relationship between us, I think, like two old friends who had quarreled.

T: Did you find that you could spend your spare moments with Rover?

P: Yes, he seemed always around, usually on the other side of the room.

T: What do you mean?

P: If I would sit and just think I could see a little black dog.

T: How real would he appear?

P: I think, pretty real.

T: Were there times when you were relating to him, that you forgot that he was just imaginary?

P: I don't know, I think so. I don't have too much spare time. I almost wish he was actual flesh and blood, I really do. Several times I thought, "How would I feel if he were actually sitting here beside me and I were stroking him?"

T: You always kept him on the other side of the room?

P: Not always. Let's put it this way, several times when I was sitting by myself and I would think of him sitting there on the other side of the room, I would wish he would come over so I could pet him and he did.

T: You could let him come over?

P: Yes, I would think how he would feel. I didn't have that reaction of cringing I have always had when I touched a dog. I think I fully wished that he were a real flesh and blood concrete thing that I could feel.

T: How do you think he felt sitting on the other side of the room?

P: Probably the same way I did, wishing we could make up. That is the feeling I have, we are like two friends who quarreled over something insignificant and don't know how to make up.

T: After 41 years you are ready to forgive him?

P: I think I should not have blamed him in the first place.

T: However, it was a natural thing for a child to do.

P: Yes, for a child. It was a funny thing to blame the dog, wasn't it? I wish I had blamed someone else so I could still have had the dog for a playmate.

T: If you had not blamed the dog, you may have ended up blaming yourself.

P: Well, yes, that's right. That would have been serious if I had thought I had actually caused my sister's death.

T: Your mother might have been able to convince you then.

P: [Long pause.] I was just thinking how interesting this profession must be. It is wonderful to be able to go back and uncover these things. I wonder if a lot of illnesses are not caused by things that happened in our earlier lives. I am probably not thinking about what I should be.

T: This time is entirely yours to do with as you wish. If the pressure of your problems is reduced so you can think of other things, maybe that is good. You seem much more relaxed today.

P: I feel much more relaxed. Of course, there were days when I was quite depressed, but I can feel myself coming out of it. I think I am returning to being a happy, normal person. Several people who often drop into the house for coffee and to talk have remarked lately that I seemed so depressed that I wasn't any use to them. They came to my house to cheer up and found out I wasn't very cheerful, so I think they will be happy when I return to normal.

T: Your usual behavior is to give support to others?

P: Yes, that seems a little odd. I wasn't too aware of it. It has always been easy to listen to others. There is always someone around a school who needs someone to listen to them. I hadn't realized how much so until they needed a dean of women last spring. I was quite amused when the girls got up a petition to make me dean. They did not know what they were asking. Two deans in one family would be quite hectic. And, of course, I would not be interested in a full-time job. But my husband was quite flattered by it, and after I got over being amused I guess I was too. But having always sort of helped with other people's problems, maybe that is why I got over mine as I have.

T: It sometimes helps to concern oneself with other's problems.

P: Yes, I think so. When we came here we knew we would be dealing with a different type of student. We had been used to dealing with students with less money than these kids, but it didn't take us long to find out that they have their problems too. I guess people everywhere have problems.

T: How do you feel about your specific problem, the fear of dogs?

P: I am so grateful we uncovered it. I think now that we have, I should be able to handle it. Not completely yet, but certainly better than I was. I can think about dogs in a different manner, the fact that I would have liked very much for my little black Harvey to be real. I was thinking the other night when I was sitting in the living room by myself, I wanted to touch him and see how he would feel. I think I could have. At least I know what I am afraid of, there isn't anything so bad as being afraid of the unknown. That's how I feel about it.

T: What if you were to find out this was all a figment of your imagination?

P: If it was, it's a mighty interesting figment. I don't think it was. Things I had completely forgotten I could verify, by letters and various data, so I know I didn't make them up. And the fact that the same process could also keep Dr. Segerson from hurting me and he hasn't ever not hurt me before, those things are to me proof. The very fact my mother remembered the little black dog, maybe she has the name wrong, but the fact remains the little black dog was there.

T: Validity lies in the fact that the things you have been able to check hold up, the intensity of the feelings associated with these memories, and the logical consistency of everything we have been able to uncover.

P: Yes, and the fact that it all makes sense to my husband, and he remembered something else. When my dad died, on the way to St. Louis, my husband said, "You know that none of your sisters and brothers are going to ask your mother to live with them; don't you think we should?" I can remember the frustration within me. I appreciated so much his graciousness in offering, but I didn't want my mother to come live with me. I didn't know why then. And I wouldn't do it unless we would actually build on to our ranch-style house a separate place of her own. I knew I have never been close to my mother but didn't know why an adult should feel that way about her mother. I was ashamed of myself.

T: Now it is not necessary to feel ashamed of yourself?

P: No, I think I know why I felt that way. We were as good to her as we could be and she lived with us one and a half years. She wasn't always happy because she didn't like to live around the college atmosphere, but that is all we could offer. Then we left there and went down to Arkansas and tried to find an apartment that was adequate for a wheelchair patient, so we bought this rambling, 12-room house just to make Mother happy. She wasn't happy and I don't think any of us were really. Then we learned she was affecting Judy. In kindergarten Judy would not admit she had a grandmother and the teacher knew she had. So she thought we had better look into it. We saw there was a great deal of resentment there.

T: Again you see how a child handles something unpleasant by denying it.

P: Yes, and we were amazed because Judy was a very outgoing girl who loved everyone. I knew there was conflict, but I thought it was the age-old conflict between age and youth but it was more than that, I guess, so we put Mother in a home. Or rather my husband explained to her that nobody was very happy in this situation so she chose to go to this home. She didn't like it and so my sister took her in her home and it didn't work there either. She had a little boy nine and the same sort of conflict seemed to enter in. I think over the years Mother has not been able to get along well with anyone.

I am going to talk to her about this. I am going into St. Louis next week and see her. Should I or shouldn't I? Not about what I am doing here, she wouldn't understand it, but what we've discovered.

T: There is a possibility she might find it disturbing.

P: Of course, I don't want that to happen. I would like to ask her if she could remember a little more about it, though. Maybe she can tell me what happened to the little black dog, if he went right away.

T: Of course, she has maintained you have been afraid of dogs all of your life, so she apparently doesn't accept the significance of the situation we uncovered.

P: Yes, she has maintained I have had this fear all my life. I remember she would get quite angry if I questioned it. An obstetrician-friend of ours says that no such thing could have happened, that children are not born with fears, they acquire them, but she believes very firmly I was born with this fear.

T: I think you would have to be very inventive in the type of questions you asked her.

P: You mean so she would give answers she didn't mean to give?

T: Something like that.

P: I wish there was someone else I could talk to. The only other one is an uncle down in southeast Missouri. Isn't it true that older people remember things more sharply later in life? I think he might remember. He was married to my Aunt Ethel.

T: Could you ask your brothers?

P: We have never been a very close family. I could talk to my brother in California, he might remember. He was about nine then. I have a brother in St. Louis I haven't seen for about four years. I don't know where he lives.

T: It's important to confirm that it happened in exactly this way?

P: No, because I believe it really did happen this way. No, it's not important except that I am one of those people who like to catalogue things.

T: What direction do you think these sessions should take now?

P: Maybe to a kennel somewhere? [Laughs.] I don't know. You are going to let me keep my little Rover, aren't you, so I can keep getting used to him?

T: Do you want him?

P: Yes, I think I will keep him.

T: He doesn't frighten you?

P: No.

T: Have you let anyone else in on our little secret?

P: No, I certainly couldn't tell Judy, she would take him away from me.

T: It is my feeling that you have made considerable progress in the several sessions we have had.

P: Well, I have worked hard.

T: I think you deserve a lot of credit for that. Now we are coming to a period when it might be best to take a break, a period in which you can continue to work on the problem and then we might meet again in a few weeks to see how you have progressed. We might set the time at a month, perhaps the 17th of March?

P: We have got to be through by April because Judy said the other night that since I had not given her a puppy for her birthday, she would give me one for mine.

T: If it's all right with you then, sit back and relax. I will give you a few suggestions to take along with you.

P: Good, I was hoping that you would. [Patient goes deeply asleep.]

T: You have worked hard the past seven sessions and I think you can see the many benefits you are reaping. The roots of this problem go deep and you can see how your ability to face your past has succeeded in improvement of your adjustment in many directions. As you mentioned today, you feel more comfortable in disciplining Judy. You have also mentioned now understanding this feeling of moral obligation felt towards members of your family. You have a better understanding of your negative feelings towards your mother and this should reduce your reaction of guilt concerning the death of your second child. Your work here should make your life still more positive, productive, and rewarding.

Regarding your fear of dogs, this was only the most obvious symptom resulting from your earlier disturbing experiences. Here, too, your fear, appropriate as a little child, is no longer appropriate today. In opening this door of memory you have opened the way to emotional growth. The little-girl side of you who remained afraid of dogs and all that fear meant now has the opportunity to grow up. Often as children we are faced by what seem to be insurmountable fears or problems and as a child we try to block them off. Years later, as an adult, we may fear that we have a bear or savage dog trapped in the closet of our unconscious. When we open the door we find that this ferocious bear may turn out to be more of a teddy bear. We have grown up and learned to handle these feelings.

In the past few days, Rover, the little black dog of your childhood, has been with you. You mentioned that you want to keep him awhile longer. Apparently you are growing in your feelings of comfort with Rover. You feel more sorry for him than dislike or fear of him. Because you are now beginning to see him with the eyes of an adult rather than a lonely, rejected little girl, I will let you keep Rover quite a bit longer, so long as you continue to work on your problems. He will be there at moments when you want to renew acquaintance with this old friend who represents your unhappy childhood. You will find it increasingly possible to shorten the physical and emotional distance between you two. This is a situation over which you have complete control: Rover can be as near or as far as you wish. He can be as far as your fear of him or as near as your new understanding will allow. You should find that in a relatively short time it will be quite comfortable to have him close beside you.

We have a date to work towards, March 17, when you will return. I am confident that between now and then you will continue to work on this problem consciously and unconsciously. Of course, it will not be possible for you to keep Rover indefinitely. As you pointed out today, it would be so nice to have Rover really there. I think you can have Rover *really there* in a sense that down through the years Rover has always been there in every dog that you met, particularly in little, frisky dogs. Each dog has been Rover as you looked at him with your little girl eyes. If you work hard at becoming friends with Rover, your fear will leave you and you will quite naturally develop a greater acceptance of all dogs. As time goes on you will develop the idea of having a real Rover for you to enjoy and especially Judy, who needs and wants a Rover of her own. I anticipate this will be the natural succession of events.

March 17 is our target date. Don't put off your homework until the last few days. If you work steadily at this problem, I am confident you will become relatively comfortable, not only with

Rover, but with all Rovers, and particularly the little Rover Judy so badly wants. I think the day you take Judy out and buy her this dog, we can consider you cured of this fear. In purchasing such a dog, the real importance will lie in the fact that you have straightened out your life, swept clean in many directions, and this dog will come to symbolize this fact. You will be demonstrating that your own unfortunate childhood experiences will not keep you from rearing Judy in a healthy fashion. After you awaken, I want you to go forward with the determination and conviction that in the next few weeks you can successfully resolve your problems. [Patient is awakened.]

P: Oh, I feel I slept so long.

T: Do you feel fairly satisfied and happy about everything?

P: I think so. I feel like this has been a very successful experience. I think I know myself better; I don't know if I like myself better, but I know myself better.

Session VIII, March 18

T: Well, now, tell me about your month.

P: Well, now, let me see . . . most of it is in here [points to manuscript she is carrying], but I will tell you anyhow. Tuesday, after I left here, I took Judy out skating and there were two or three puppy dogs. It seemed very natural to reach down and pet them, there was no fear of doing it. It didn't feel like dogs used to feel, I felt amused, I did it unconsciously. I heard Judy yell, "Oh, look, Mommy used to be afraid of dogs and isn't anymore." Then it dawned on me, well, I really wasn't. That was the 18th, I believe. It seemed right after that I lost Rover. You don't have him around here anymore, do you?

T: I haven't seen him.

P: Well, he isn't around, I guess he was jealous and he left me. I thought of him continuously until that day. He sort of left me after that and I had a hard time thinking about him.

This weekend we went home and I was sorry the dog was gone. I wanted to see how I would react to that dog. Mother James said he had left about a week ago. I almost said he and Rover ran off together but I didn't. Judy found another little animal in the neighborhood which she brought home. It was very easy for me to pet him, and I didn't feel the way I had before.

They are still looking for a dog. In fact, I didn't know they were looking. My husband was gone all last week and someone called, that I did not recognize, and I took a message. He said, "Look, tell Mr. James that the dog will not be available until around May." I didn't know he was looking for a dog, but I guess he is. So, we are going to have a dog.

T: Are you reconciled to it?

P: Well, yes, I don't know why we haven't been able to pick a dog up yet, but I think I could. What happened way back there that gave me a recoil when I touched a dog seemed connected with my sister's death, didn't it? What happened?

T: Do you remember discussing how you felt about touching a dog?

P: No, I wasn't ever afraid the dog would bite me, I just didn't want it to come running at me. If the dog was over there and I knew it would stay over there, I was all right but if I thought it would come over and I would have to touch it, it would bother me. I didn't want to touch it or have him touch me. So, apparently, there was something in my realizing she was dead. There must have been something in connection with the way she felt, don't you imagine?

T: I would assume so.

P: Another interesting thing happened to me. I visited my Uncle Earl, Aunt Ethel's husband, he is 86 now and we talked quite a while. He couldn't remember an incident like this having happened, but he said he was not at our house until the time of the funeral, but he did seem to remember rather definitely that I wasn't afraid of dogs until that time. He also remembered that we had a little black dog. Another interesting thing, I asked him what the inside of our house looked like, because I couldn't remember and he described it as I had seen it. The way the room, in which my sister was, was off the main room. I asked him where the woodpile was in the yard, and he said it was in the rear which is where I seem to have seen it. He couldn't remember this incident; then I remembered that about this time he was rather a gay blade, and I doubt that anyone would have told him about it. He was drinking quite heavily at the time. I expect he was not told about it. I thought it was significant that he remembered about the little black dog and the way he described the interior of the house.

Then, I got the picture from my sister and I had her find the one I knew had been taken with myself and two dogs. I remember disliking that picture very much. They were both little black dogs.

Someone was holding the dogs, however. I had a gun in my arms, so I guess they knew they better hold those dogs. I remember having my picture made when I was about five. The picture was made at my grandfather's farm shortly before I left. Probably one of them was the dog in question. My husband thought, since there were two dogs that looked exactly alike, one of them might have been the dog I thought was Rover and the other the one that Mother remembers as Twister. They looked exactly alike.

At least I don't feel the same way about dogs and I am anxious to get that puppy to see how I feel about him. I told the man on the phone that I hoped it would be black. He said, "What did you say?" and I told him it didn't matter. Of course, I don't know too much about dogs. I have never been very interested in them. Preston said something about a Shepherd. There is a cute, little Cocker Spaniel tied outside the Seminole Apartments; I would like to know whose he is. It has the most interesting little face.

T: How do you feel about this whole process?

P: It has been very fascinating. Probably the most exciting thing, or one of the most exciting things, that has ever happened to me.

T: It was certainly a unique opportunity to go back and explore into the past.

P: Yes, do people do it often?

T: Yes, with some frequency but usually it is spread over a much longer period of time. It depends on the individual's ability to face up to the past.

P: I think I have a rather unique ability to face up to almost anything. I felt there was something there, but I had no way of finding it. I thought someday I would meet someone who could help me find it.

T: How much faith do you have that these memories are substantially correct? As you recall, you questioned this the last time.

P: I am the type of person who likes proof of everything. The way Mother and Uncle Earl recall certain things, it couldn't all be incorrect. I know we had dogs up until the time my little sister died, so it all seems that it must be so. Did my mind make up something like this?

T: The main thing I am questioning here is your attitude towards this memory.

P: It seems to me it must be so, since part of it can be verified. Let's say this, if it is not correct, I will accept it because it has changed my feeling towards dogs.

T: You feel fairly confident that when the dog arrives, you will be able to take him in stride?

P: If I am not, I will be here the next day [laughs]. I really do though. I felt so differently about these dogs that I petted and touched. Whether the incident is true or false, my attitude has changed.

T: You can see these dogs more realistically now?

P: Yes, I always knew that I felt about them like a child but there was nothing I could do about it, I just couldn't. I tried but I just couldn't! When a dog would come near me and I would touch it, I would actually shudder. So there must have been something early in my life to cause that.

T: This reaction you are describing held right up until the time you came here?

P: Oh, yes. When we came here Preston got Judy a pup to help her adjust. I wondered if he thought what he was doing to my adjustment. I managed to hold it one day to take its picture but I actually trembled all over. It took all the courage I had and some I didn't have. I was always afraid of the dog and I think it knew it. When I came home from class, I was scared to death that he would meet me on the campus. I had this feeling right up to the time I came here.

T: I am interested in what you did with Rover.

P: I am too. Was he jealous because I petted the other dog? Why couldn't I think of him anymore? I thought about him almost constantly from the time of the last session until last Tuesday, in a friendly way, I guess. After the incident in which I petted the puppy, I couldn't force myself to think about him, I would try but I couldn't. I wonder why? Where did he go? In the first place, where did he come from?

T: He seemed quite real to you?

P: Well, yes. At least I thought about him all the time.

T: Could you see him?

P: Yes, I could.

T: Did you tell your husband about him?

P: No, but he read about him in here [in her manuscript] and he didn't say a word about it. I guess he thought like I felt — that this was worse than he thought it was.

T: Seeing him frightened you somewhat at first?

P: Yes, but I don't know where he went but he isn't around anymore.

T: Do you think he outlived his usefulness and is now finding a rest?

P: I kind of think so. And then I dreamed about a dog, it was different. It did not have any horror or fear. There was a large dog leaning against me and he felt more like a child leaning against me. I had that dream sometime around the 18th.

T: Your fear of dogs has not been a problem for the past several weeks?

P: No, it has not been a problem since the 18th.

T: Since Rover left, you have had a comfortable feeling about dogs?

P: Yes, I think I could go to anyone's house now without even considering whether they had a dog or not. I don't think I would be at all afraid now.

The patient and therapist then exchanged manuscripts. The patient handed over a 59-page narration concerning her feelings and reactions during therapy. The therapist gave her a complete transcription of the seven preceding sessions.

P: Did you tell me to write this? It all came so easily. Even the sequence of events came so easily.

T: I didn't tell you to do this directly but it may have been implied to you consciously and unconsciously in the instructions given you during your sessions.

P: Perhaps that was it.

It was agreed that patient and therapist would read each other's manuscripts and would meet again in one week to discuss them.

Session IX, March 24

T: What did you think of the transcription of the sessions?

P: It was most interesting.

T: Were you surprised by anything you read?

P: Yes, I was. Some things I did not remember and some things I remember vaguely. Yes, there were some surprises.

T: I certainly enjoyed reading your own story.

P: I was a little embarrassed about coming back to see you today after I had remarked that your chair was not comfortable [laughs].

I thought it was a very interesting experience. I certainly derived benefits in a lot of ways. I mentioned that my husband never talked about the children we had lost. It was never mentioned until I came here. Last night he was reading the Sunday magazine section of the *Post-Dispatch* and he remarked that a picture reminded him of Penny, the little girl we had lost. He said it so naturally, there was not the reserve which I am sure had always been there before. I had surprised him by having her picture made the second day after she was born. The picture in the paper was of a new-born baby and looked very much like our little girl. I though it was good he could mention it without reservation. I thought about that as one of the gains that had come from this.

T: I tend to feel that anything you can talk about, you can begin to accept.

P: I know it must have hurt him terribly to lose three children, but I don't know what made him so quiet unless he felt as I did that it would only hurt the other by talking about it, but he never mentioned it and last night it was just a natural offhand remark. I was glad that he could speak of it that way. That is not at all the reason I came here, but I am glad that came about too.

T: I think you have an awareness that no problem occurs in isolation and that we discussed a lot of things which on the surface had not seemed related. I notice in the manuscript that you state there are other things that you experienced but did not want to talk about.

P: Yes, but they were not important. I am sure they were not. Now you are not going to hypnotize me and get me to tell you all these things are you [laughs]? Really, there is no relationship, I am sure. I see no reason why I even remembered them except that I was remembering everything apparently. Is it customary for patients to have to remember everything and especially in a chronological order?

T: I would say that a great many people are not as thorough in their housecleaning as you are.

P: Well, it seemed like I had to do an awful lot. It was interesting especially since there were so many things which I had forgotten. I think it was good too, even all the dates I remembered, because if anyone had asked me I would have said, "Oh, yes, I had dates." But my sister was the belle of the ball and I did not want to be.

T: You were surprised to find that you were more popular than you had remembered yourself as being?

P: Much more so. I was shocked when I mentioned to my husband the different men I had dated. I knew in college I had quite an inferiority complex but I did not know until later how severe it really was and certainly not completely until all this came up. I don't think I have much now, although I may have more than I know. Saturday there were some people at our home and I remarked that 10 years ago I could not have talked at the High School Career Day, I just could not have. There were surprised I had ever been like that. They could not imagine I had ever felt that way.

T: It was in such contrast to the way they see you now.

P: Yes, they did not know me then. They just could not believe that I had been so shy with people. I don't think I am that way now, really. I don't think it matters now what people think. I am that uninhibited.

T: That is a good index of security.

P: I think I feel secure now.

T: In reference to the material you don't want to talk about, let me assure you that it is not necessary for you to talk about everything.

P: No, I think not and if I felt there were anything important there, I would.

T: You certainly have a right to your privacy. How have you felt the last couple of sessions about our relationship?

P: I feel less like a patient. In fact, about three weeks ago we had something up at the college and Preston said wouldn't it be nice to have Dr. and Mrs. Moss out to dinner and I said, "No, not now. I would feel too much like a patient." But, I don't feel that way now. I think I would like to know you socially now.

T: I had seen you undergoing this change and wondered about it.

P: Yes, I feel differently about it.

T: I have the impression that you felt that this problem was pretty well resolved, that much of the original motivation had been spent. I also had the impression that you are anxious to get this over with.

P: I think it is characteristic that when I do anything I am in a hurry to get it over with and get on to something else.

T: How near completion or solution do you think the problem is?

P: I don't know. What do you think about it?

T: We learn to be cautious in this type of work but it seems to me there are many indications that the end is near.

P: Yes, I know I feel entirely different about it. I had a dream last night. I was visiting in someone's home, a fabulous home, so it was obviously a dream and they had two little puppies. They quite fascinated me. They were little honey-colored puppies, not black. I could hardly talk to the gentleman. I do not know who he was. I seemed to be a friend of the woman. I was talking to him about the dogs. Where he got them and if he thought I could get some. He assured me I could. We were sitting by the table. One of them touched my leg. I had always hated to be touched by a dog. My first impulse was to put my feet in the chair but then I thought, "This is silly because I am not afraid of dogs anymore." It did not feel awful like it used to. I thought it was interesting that I should dream of them especially since I had only been thinking about black dogs.

Then on Monday night the man across the street brought his little dog over, the one who is so active and is kept on a leash all the time. He called and asked if he could bring it over. I wanted to see how I would react to the dog. It was the most active dog I have ever seen. I think, in fact, if it was let loose it would climb the wall, it is that kind of dog. I didn't like its activeness, it worried me. I talked to Preston about it afterwards. He said he didn't think my reaction was much worse than his or Judy's, as much as Judy likes dogs. She doesn't like a dog to jump all over her. So I was glad to know he thought I had not reacted too abnormally. I didn't want the man to turn him loose in the house and he didn't either, so I guess I didn't act too differently from Preston. I thought about it all today, and was disappointed I could not wholeheartedly accept the active dog but then he didn't and Judy didn't so I guess it was all right. The only time the dog was the least bit intimidated was when Judy tried to take it upstairs. It was afraid of the stairs and it was quiet then. I think I was more irked that it would not be still so I could pet it.

T: You have some better understanding of what it is about the feel of a dog which you find disturbing?

P: Yes, I think so.

T: Did you read the section in which we had discussed this?

P: Yes, oddly enough I had forgotten that.

T: I think you would find that even if you had not read the transcription that a good many of these details would come back later on. You might not recognize they had been gone into here, though.

P: It is a funny thing. What if I had retained that fear of touching a
dead person, as much contact as I have had with dead people in
my life? I know a lot more than the average person about this.
Something like that happened at the college last week. A girl died
and her roommate had never been that close to death before and
was very upset. I don't think it left me with any fear of death, I
cannot remember ever being afraid of death itself.

T: You did remark that your sister's death had given you a greater
acceptance of it.

P: Yes, but I think it was an acceptance in a different way. I wasn't
afraid of it before; I thought about it differently after that, however.

T: Did your husband read the transcription?

P: Yes, we thought it most interesting. He was sitting over there
chuckling and I asked him what he was laughing about. He said,
"Well, that little dog he gave you, I think that was a real good trick
on you." He thought it was quite interesting.

T: Did you come to any increased understanding as to why Rover
left you?

P: Yes, I think he doesn't need to be around anymore. I hope I am
not kidding myself. I think that is why. The mind sure does funny
things, doesn't it? There are two or three points in there which I
did not understand. One place I kept saying that my mother
blamed me for my sister's death as a small child, when I told her
that I missed my sister. I did not remember having told you that
or ever even feeling that way. It surprised me it was in there. There
was one point in there in which I actually said I missed my sister
and she told me it was my fault she was gone. I did not think I had
told you that or I didn't remember that it had ever happened. That
was the only important point that I can think of.

T: It is still seemingly difficult for you to accept that all of this happened in every detail. I might say that in reading your manuscript
I was impressed with the clarity with which you express yourself.
Once I got into it, I found that your phrasing caused it to move
right along.

P: I don't know, that's the way it came to me. I don't think I usually
write that way. When my husband read it, he thought it was not
always clear. Something very funny happened which I think you
will get a kick out of. On the way home from Uncle Earl's the
other day, I was talking about Uncle Earl having described the interior of our house and which I didn't remember. And yet he de-

scribed it as I saw it in hypnosis. Without thinking I said, "Well, I am going to ask Dr. Moss if that's the way he remembers it." Preston got a big kick out of that. For a moment I forgot that you were not there with me. He thought that was quite rare.

T: It is interesting how hypnosis reduces the distinction between objective and subjective.

P: Yes, very definitely.

T: I guess little else remains to be done until the first of May.

P: The first of May? I may not be able to wait that long. I may go to Beloit to a pet show there.

T: It does seem a shame now that you are in the mood for a dog that you have to wait.

P: Yes, I am afraid I might change my mind or something.

T: Does it almost seem too good to be true?

P: Yes, I think so. I don't think Judy wants to wait until then either. There must be a pet shop in Beloit. I don't know of any in Madison.

T: I think it would be nice if you could select a dog that particularly appeals to you.

P: Yes, I think so too. I was so sure I wanted a little black Cocker Spaniel but that was a cute yellow dog I dreamed about last night. I am going over to Beloit Wednesday. I might do some checking while I am over there.

T: What reservations do you have now about the use of this material?

P: I think none.

T: I don't know how I will use this material, if I will at all, but knowing about it might provide courage or confidence for people who have similar problems.

P: It seems like a subject that is rather timely now. I don't know, after I wrote it all down and sat and thought about it, there is a lot of my personal life in there. I would certainly want my identity hidden.

T: I think if it were ever published in any form, you should have the opportunity to go over it. You can see from your experience with *The Three Faces of Eve*, the value in making this type of thing public.

P: Yes, but oddly enough though, many, many years before I wished I could meet somebody when we were in west Texas and very good friends of the doctors on the staff there. I talked to them about a psychiatrist there at the hospital, but he was an odd sort of person. I remember one of the surgeons said, "Pauline, I think I would wait and go someplace else." He said that he thought this doctor was a victim of his own profession. So I thought about it a long time ago. I knew it was something I could not handle. I guess that was the only other real chance I had until we came here. I read *Three Faces of Eve* first: after having read it I thought there *is* somebody who can help me with this and I wondered how I could go about finding someone. I was very glad to meet you. After having gone through this I felt that there are many people like me who have talked to me about the "somethings" in their life. It is not an uncommon thing. I think that is why I wrote it down and thought somebody might read it and be encouraged to seek help.

On April 6, the patient phoned to say that she had purchased a small dog, a black Cocker Spaniel, whom she had named Happy Siesta. She confessed wanting to name it after the therapist but hesitated to do so in fear that he might be offended. Therefore, she incorporated his first two initials into a name.[9]

February 11

A brief followup session was held. There was evidence that repressive forces were still active, in that her memory of the events discussed in therapy was somewhat faulty and she stated that some aspects of her recall were "not quite real." She also reported that while her mother had continued to deny that the event had ever happened, she was in possession of two additional bits of confirmatory evidence. A brother recalled the existence of Rover and the fact that she and her sister had been left temporarily alone at the time of the accident due to a fire at a neighbor's house across the road; and her younger sister confirmed that as children the patient had always anxiously protected her in the presence of all dogs. She reaffirmed that therapy had somewhat altered her family relationships, but the most evident effect of therapy continued to be a basic change in her attitude toward

---

[9] It is possible this name is overdetermined; it could also refer to the hypnotic experience, or at a deeper level, a euphemistic expression representing her reconciliation to death.

dogs: "All my life the touch of a dog gave me a feeling of something horrible — I'm still surprised that I feel so differently now."

DISCUSSION

This case provides a clear demonstration of the use of psychotherapeutic procedure in modification of a long-standing learning process. Adjunctive hypnotic techniques were of especial value in rapidly uncovering and revivifying the childhood pathogenic experience, allowing the person to grapple with it in a new attempt at mastery. Relearning was facilitated by reinstatement on a symbolic fantasy level of the patient's relationship with the original object of her phobia and with sufficient vividness to make it a realistic and immediate emotional experience.

Hypnosis was also of value in reinforcing the patient's motivational level and at times in providing an almost compulsive re-experiencing of long-forgotten memories. In this manner, substantial progress was facilitated between sessions and following the termination of formal sessions, apparently significantly shortening the period of actual treatment. Success in this direct relearning procedure was naturally dependent on the assessed capacity of the patient's ego to assimilate repressed infantile experiences into conscious awareness.

The foundation for the patient's neurosis appears to have been a lack of understanding, acceptance, and emotional warmth in relation to her parents, particularly the mother. The traumatic incident in which she was unjustly accused of her sister's death focused her feelings of being mistreated, misunderstood, and rejected onto dogs. Specifically, the physical sensation of her sister's cold, still body became associated with its opposite, the warmth and liveliness of the real culprit, her dog. In a sense, dogs thus became an idiosyncratic symbol of the disturbed relationship with her mother.

In spite of her use of the dog as an object for projection and her protestations of innocence, continued accusation and rejection by her mother seem to have generated some guilt in the patient. This guilt appeared in her eagerness for punishment as a child, which may be variously interpreted as direct atonement, as assertion of innocence by being unjustly punished (a repetition of the circumstances surrounding her sister's death), as a technique for forcing her mother to support her innocence by having continuously to get her out of trouble, or all of these. Some feelings of guilt were also apparent in the deaths of her children, and it appeared very important for her to prove to her husband that she was not to blame.

One important consequence seems to have been the patient's inability to express directly her feelings of hostility and resentment. A hypothesis that had to be considered during treatment was that she originally had projected these feelings onto her dog and that her phobia protected against their expression. Her desire to present her daughter with a puppy (dependent on eradication of the "protective" symptom) might then have negative implications. Fortunately, the year witnessed some improvement in the patient's relationship with her daughter with no evidence of an increased display of hostility.

The approach employed encouraged the patient to re-evaluate the influence of her childhood experiences in terms of present-day understanding and to effect a fuller readjustment, not only to the original conflict but to its ramifications in her present-day life. No claim is made for achievement of a complete cure in the sense that the patient achieved full readjustment to all aspects of the widely generalized effect of the original conflict. Neither should the impression be conveyed that hypnotherapeutic techniques afforded a panacea per se. The patient described her youth as characterized by "a fear of people, new situations, many things" and her marriage as having had a highly therapeutic effect. The death of a beloved older sister when the patient was age 27 helped the patient partially overcome her fear of death. Factors such as these contributed to a substantial degree of "spontaneous recovery" and established a "readiness" to circumvent the repressive defense upon which the hypnotherapeutic procedure then capitalized.

The objective measurement of changes concomitant with psychotherapy always provides an important challenge to the clinician. In this study use was again made of the semantic differential, a versatile instrument developed for the measurement of the feeling aspects of meaning. Factor analysis of judgments of the concept ME by 100 subjects, reported in *The Measurement of Meaning* (Osgood et al., 1957), yielded six suggestive independent factors. More recently a new differential based on the framework provided by these provisional factors was constructed. Three clearly defined and stable factors were found: "morality" (analogue of the general evaluation factor); "volatility" (analogue of the general activity factor); and "toughness" (analogue of the usual potency factor). Three additional factors were suggested. It is now proposed to clarify this "personality factor structure" using new scales, subjects, concepts, and factor analysis. It is then planned to test the stability of this system in a variety of situations where personality descriptions are typically made, e.g., in describing personalities as revealed in job or clinical interviews. It is hoped there can eventually be developed a short form differential (no more than 18 scales) that can serve as a standardized instrument for describing the "personality" of self or others in a wide range of situations.

In this study the patient was requested to rate six concepts on a six-factor [10] form of the semantic differential at the first session, to repeat these ratings at the seventh session (last formal contact), then one month and again at one year after termination. She was also asked to periodically rate the concept ROVER after his existence was discovered during the fourth session. A

---

[10] The scales employed represent six factors (inferred meaning): dependability (dependable-undependable, sober-drunk, moral-immoral); dominance (straight-curved, hard-soft, strong-willed–weak-willed); volatility (excitable-calm, changeable-stable, emotional-unemotional); individuality (colorful-colorless, interesting-boring, striking-plain); sociability (outgoing–self-centered, sociable-unsociable, open-closed); structuredness (formed-formless, real-unreal, shallow-deep).

comparison of the quantitative alterations in meaning experienced by the patient in relation to these concepts is represented in Table 13.

TABLE 13. Comparison in terms of distance statistic (D) of over-all quantitative changes in meaning of seven concepts.

Concept	Ratings		
	I:II	I:III	I:IV
CATS	3.46	4.24	4.36
DOGS	3.00	5.88	7.07
SELF	5.10	6.93	6.56
MOTHER	5.74	8.12	7.94
FATHER	4.47	6.16	7.07
THERAPIST	4.36	6.48	5.92
ROVER	—	7.87	7.55

I = first session; II = last formal session; III = one-month followup; IV = 12-month followup.

It is apparent that the meaning of ROVER changed considerably, especially when contrasted to the control concept CATS. As would be anticipated, changes in meaning of this central concept ROVER apparently generalized, resulting in an altered meaning of dogs in general. A substantial change in attitude toward the parents is also evidenced (see Fig. 19).

The major changes in meaning occurred on the factors of dependability, volatility, and structuredness. There was a consistent tendency to rate concepts as better formed and more real, perhaps reflecting greater clarity of perception. A summary of the qualitative alterations in meaning relative to each concept rated follows.

ROVER. When first remembered, Rover was considered undependable, unsocial, immoral, and somewhat unreal. Later he was perceived as soft, curved, more sociable, real, neither moral nor immoral, and definitely colorful and interesting.

DOGS. Seen originally as very changeable, strong-willed, and excitable; later perceived (like ROVER) as much more colorful and interesting, soft, sociable, and real.

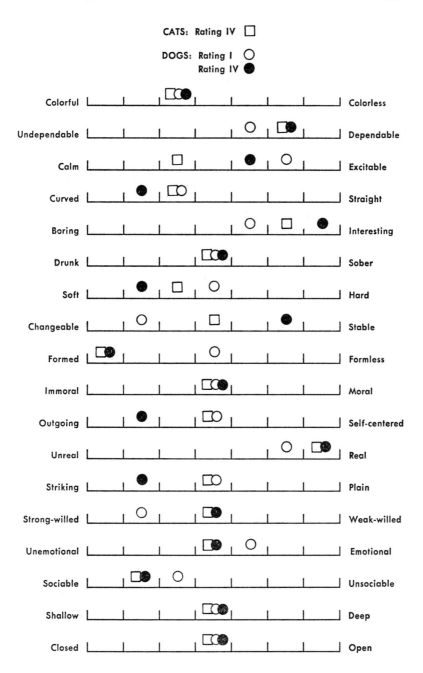

FIG. 19. Contrast of ratings on the semantic differential over time.

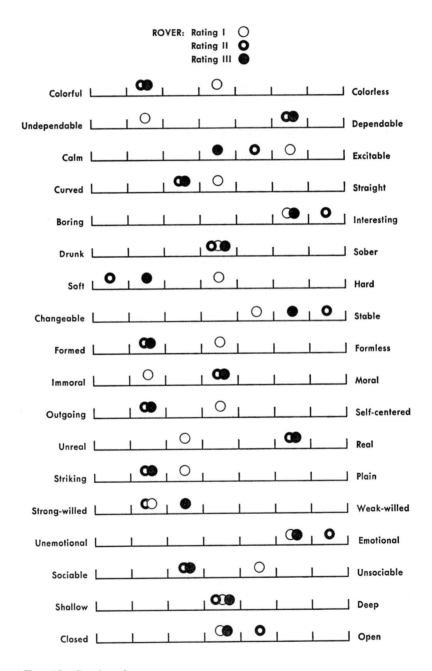

Fig. 19. *Continued.*

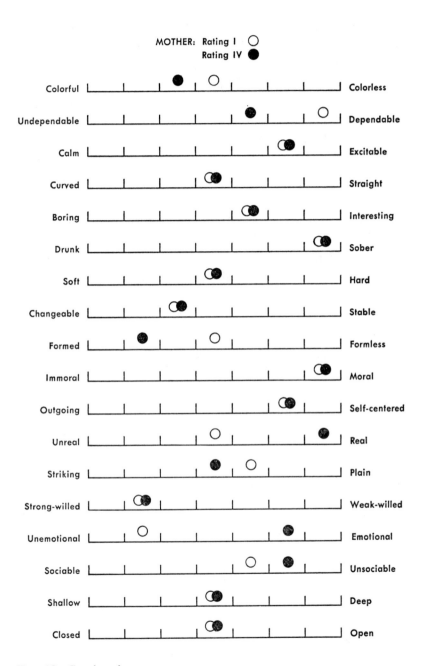

FIG. 19. *Continued.*

HAPPY SIESTA. Rated only at time of terminal followup interview as extremely colorful, interesting, dependable, soft, stable, outgoing, sociable, formed, and real.

CATS. Seen rather consistently as colorful, dependable, soft, real, and sociable; also as less excitable, weaker-willed, and slightly less outgoing than DOGS.

FATHER. Described initially as dependable, calm, interesting, moral, real, sociable, and slightly weak-willed. In followup interviews he was rated as more excitable and emotional, less sober and stable.

MOTHER. Originally described as somewhat dependable, excitable, changeable, self-centered, and unsociable, very sober, moral, and strong-willed. In the final ratings she was seen as less dependable, sober, hard, and self-centered, and more sociable, real, and formed.

SELF. Patient pictured self as very dependable, moral, rather calm, stable, outgoing, and sociable, and slightly colorless. Final ratings showed few sizable shifts aside from thinking of herself as more formed, real, and stronger-willed.

THERAPIST. Consistently perceived as dependable, calm, interesting, stable, moral, outgoing, and strong-willed. Largest changes were in the direction of rating him as more formed, real, and less sober.

Five years after the final 12-month followup (August, 1966) the patient responded to an inquiry by the therapist.

I apologize for the delay but I am involved in new duties at the school which seem to consume a lot of time. And I have probably spent too much time enjoying the pool. At any time I could help you further with this I shall be happy to do so.

The fear of dogs has never returned. I still do not like to have dogs jump up on me but I believe this is a normal reaction. It does not come from fear but a desire to save hosiery and clothes. My daughter still has a dog, and I am certainly not afraid of him. I am not aware of any new fears that might have replaced the old one. In fact, I think I am generally less afraid of most things than are most people. I think

I might be less inhibited than most people. I used to be quite shy. This doesn't sound like a statement from a shy person, does it?

I have wondered about this many times. I wish I had some proof of the validity of the memories. Since this is not possible I prefer to think they were distortions. Although I haven't looked at the transcript for years, I did read it several times immediately following the sessions. Maybe I was checking up on myself. At the time I think I would have preferred a copy of the tape. I'm not sure I have a concise notion about hypnosis. Maybe I think of it as a relaxed looking deep inside oneself. Looking deeper than one could do without the help of someone trained in guiding the introspection.

One learns to be cautious concerning the objective validity of retrospective content elicited in psychotherapy, particularly when hypnosis has been employed. The fabricated memories of "Bridey Murphy" are a dramatic example of falsification. Experiments in time progression also demonstrate the vivid, realistic fantasies manufactured by hypnotized subjects. What is the evidence that this patient actually had an experience of the type she reports? Three people who might have verified her story are dead (the father, older sister, and her Aunt Ethel). The mother completely denies the whole story and has always blamed the patient's fear on prenatal influence. However, the patient recalls, and her two brothers verified the fact, that the family had several dogs prior to the time the patient was four and only the one thereafter. The patient had also remembered the "guilt identification game" but not the circumstances, while her mother has always denied this event in its entirety.

Circumstantial evidence supporting the uncovered memory is as follows. First, an uncle verified the patient's detailed recall of the house in which they had lived at the time and from which they had moved when the patient was five. Second, a sister provided a photograph of the patient at about age five standing fearfully beside a dog fitting the description of Rover. Third, a brother verified the fact that they had momentarily left the patient and her sister alone in the yard when a fire broke out at a neighbor's across the road. Fourth, relatively recent memories (within the past 20 years) were verified by the meticulous daily log and letter file kept by the patient's husband. Another type of evidence is that age regression from the time of the reported event indicated that repression occurred within months of the traumatic experience. Age regression also revealed no other basis for the patient's intense fear.

Convincing is the fact that the recovered memory logically explains many aspects of the patient's behavior: her chronic phobic reaction (especially to small, frisky dogs); her childhood need to solicit punishment, her strong fear of rejection, and a proneness to feel misunderstood; an intense ambivalence regarding her mother; a fear of unjustly disciplining her daughter, etc. Most convincing is a congruence of the known dynamic structure basic to many phobic reactions; that is, the phobia dates from an intense fear-provoking episode in childhood involving a severe disturbance of the parent-child relationship. Feelings of guilt, shame, and anxiety result in suppression and eventual repression of the frightening experience, leaving only the residual phobic symptom.

In the final analysis, the patient's loss of her phobic reaction is not wholly acceptable evidence for the validity of her recovered memories, though it may be argued that from a therapeutic point of view it makes little difference whether such an event really happened or not. For whatever reason, she has been symptom-free for more than nine years from a disruptive fear which preoccupied her for almost 40 years.

TEN

Clinical Aspects
of Hypnosymbolism

THE RELATION OF HYPNOSYMBOLIC
TREATMENT TO PSYCHOANALYSIS

In the final analysis this book was written for practicing psychotherapists as well as researchers. Freud originally placed great value on insight as a means of freeing the patient from the tyranny of the unconscious, but in time psychoanalysts were forced to admit that the treatment situation was more complicated. It is possible to effect radical changes in behavior without insight, for instance in child therapy, and similarly, it is possible to achieve insight without resulting behavioral change, as within the obsessive-compulsive. For the past 35 years, there has been decreasing emphasis on the curative effect of insight or making the unconscious conscious. Insight into infantile repression was replaced by a focus on the doctor-patient relationship — analysis of transference made therapy a living emotional experience. Attention also turned to analysis of the ego defenses.

Today many therapists emphasize that emotionally corrective experiences must precede and lay the basis for insight. Insight thus becomes an index of improvement rather than its cause; that is, "emotional insight" (as opposed to "intellectual insight") is a barometer indicating that emotional changes have already occurred. It is a matter of the efficacy of interpretation by the therapist vs. providing a safe, secure place that leads the patient to make emotionally corrective experiences. Knowledge that the historical roots of a problem are not sufficient to produce a cure nevertheless does have some value in establishing continuity in a patient's life and seemingly results in increased assimilative ability of the person through mastery of the earlier traumas.

There are a number of areas where hypnosymbolism deviates from psychoanalytic treatment in addition to being a short-term psychotherapy.

1) The heart of psychoanalytic therapy is the analysis of transference — other schools do not offer as complete analysis of the doctor-patient relationship as do the classical Freudians. The transference element, which is considered absolutely crucial in psychoanalysis, is largely ignored or minimized in hypnosymbolic treatment. This is due in part to the fact that patients are seen only for a short period of time, and usually the transference hasn't had time to really develop. Hypnosymbolic therapy is not a superficial intellectual affair, however. It is recognized that the greater the degree of neurotic involvement, the greater is the potential for distortion of present events in terms of the past. Instead, the reality of the feelings expressed in terms of the patient's dreams and fantasies are used to capture the distortion in his perceptions and to correct them. More will be said on this subject later.

2) While the therapist directly sets the stage through hypnosis for the production of dreaming and/or fantasizing, he is careful to be completely nondirective about the symbols utilized by the patient and their interpretation. First, he seldom knows what the symbols actually mean and really is dependent on the patient's interpretation. Second, he is aware that the typical dream is figuratively a projection for the subject and literally a projective stimulus for him — it is very akin to a Rorschach ink blot — and he deliberately shies away from projecting his interpretations

onto it. Third, he recognizes that the essence of hypnosymbolic treatment is in how his patient deals with it.

3) Symbolism is always regarded by the hypnotherapist as unique to the individual rather than having anything like a universal quality. It is simply unsafe for the therapist to assume that a threatening snake, for example, even in the dreams of an attractive young woman, means a penis. It could stem from an actual conditioned fear of snakes!

4) Whereas Freud valued dreams as providing access to the infantile sources of conflict and placed demand upon patients for a *linear* type of free association leading back to the infantile substructure, the hypnotic therapist, employs a *radial* type of association to amplify the immediate meaning of each dream element. This altered method of "free" association was originally delineated by Jung. Freud asked, "What is the dream caused by?" Jung asked, "What does the dream mean?" In parallel fashion the hypnotherapist asks, "What are the consequences of these symbols for the life of the client now and in the future?"

5) Finally, the hypnotherapist also acknowledges the differences between objective and subjective methods of dream interpretation. Relating the dream to situations or persons external to the dream is interpretation on the objective level; acceptance of dream images as reflective of the internal psychic situation of the dreamer is interpretation on the subjective level. It makes perfect sense to interpret symbols on either level, of course, but one is repeatedly struck by the fact that hypnotized subjects are capable of making both interpretations. For example, José fantasizes that the therapist (on *his* instructions) accompanies her going up a flight of stairs; later she confesses that the figure was actually her "masculine self" and not the therapist. Again, José dreams that she is looking for a lost skirt, and eventually she realizes the chaos in the room represents the clutter of her own mind. Free association under hypnosis tends to suspend conventional conceptual frames of reference and symbol meanings take on a very personalized self-reference.

FACTORS IN HYPNOSYMBOLISM

There is a widespread assumption that hypnotizability is a stable and consistent trait, although numerous studies that have attempted to identify the personality correlates of the "good" hypnotic subject over the last 50 years have produced negative, contradictory, and inconclusive results. The very real possibility exists that susceptibility may be more situation-specific than has been generally recognized, and the reason that no personality traits have been identified is that hypnosis can probably be induced in all normal persons under suitable conditions. Hypnotic induction cannot be divorced from hypnotic susceptibility, of course, and the usual method contains four fundamental features: first, there is a limitation of sensory intake and motor output; then comes a fixation of attention; next comes some form of repetition of monotonous stimulation; and finally, the whole process is defined as hypnosis to the subject. However, there are many exceptions to the method (including many "related states") and while each of these is *sufficient*, none of them is really a *necessary* condition.

At the same time let us admit that hypnotic induction has nothing mystical or magical about it, despite the aura that still surrounds it. Hypnotherapists generally acknowledge that the exact nature of what they say or do in the induction procedure is not as important as the "set" or expectancy of the subject to experience hypnosis. As soon as the subject has volunteered for hypnosis he is committing himself to cooperate in the procedure. Experience teaches the hypnotist that he can simplify and streamline his induction procedure to a remarkable degree. Knowing that subjects volunteer with a readiness to respond, he does not want to do or say too much to interfere with their rapid entry into hypnosis. In 1895, Breuer and Freud reported in their first casebook, *Studies in Hysteria*, that through the employment of hypnosis, they were reputedly able to demonstrate the causal connection between hysterical symptoms and unfortunate childhood experiences.

In the case of Lucie R., Freud finally met with failure in the effort to induce hynosis, with the important consequence of freeing him from dependence on this technique. He had already observed that even in hypnosis patients were sometimes resistant to frank discussion. Forced to consider alternative approaches, Freud recalled Bernheim's demonstration that the subjects' recollection of their experiences while hypnotized is only apparently forgotten in the waking state, and that such memories are immediately recoverable at the insistence of the hypnotist. He concluded that his patients really did know everything of significance and all that was necessary was to force them to impart it. Freud substituted the "trick" of placing his hands on a patient's head and asserting with great conviction that "through the pressure of my hands it will come to mind!" To his astonishment this simple maneuver enabled patients to produce much of the same content previously thought accessible only in hypnosis (Moss, 1965, pp. 11–12).

Freud never returned to the use of hypnosis. In his autobiography (1963) he identified the factors which led to his abandonment as the fact that he found that he had constantly to maintain his rapport with the patient or "even the most brilliant results were liable to be suddenly wiped away," and an experience which showed him that his patients were strongly and personally motivated, i.e., a female patient awoke and attempted to seduce him. Seduction could be a feature of the hypnotic state, as it is in all other forms of psychotherapy. Freud still could have been correct — hypnosis may be nothing more than an extremely elaborated placebo effect in which the demands of the therapist take on a heightened potency. Spelling it out most parsimoniously, the induction method may simply be a highly elaborated relaxation-sleep ritual which enables the patient to relax, to reduce his defenses, and to discard the logical syntactic rules governing thought and speech in the normal waking state. On the other hand, it all comes back to the lack of agreement as to the nature of hypnosis. To regard hypnosis as an entity may be as gross a form of simplistic thinking as was demonstrated to exist when sleep was regarded as a unitary entity. The term "hypnosis" could cover a spectrum of altered states of psychophysiological functioning, and the exact relationship between night dreams and the hypnotic state remains to be spelled out.

What is the essence of hypnosymbolic treatment? Most experts agree that hypnosis minimizes the defenses of the patient, especially the defense of repression. It does so because of a state of consciousness brought about by the special quality of the interpersonal relationship between the patient and therapist. Patient and therapist are initially in a state of unqualified positive rapport, and while in time, through the analysis of the neurotic component in the patient's personality, the relationship may become more ambivalent, the emphasis on the positive rapport is not lost, or if it is, at that juncture the person becomes resistant to hypnosis. People in hypnosis, therefore, lose some of the ability to be reflectively aware, and self-reactions of embarrassment, guilt, and anxiety are reduced. The attention of the patient is turned inward and there is accessibility to deep, emotional material of which the individual is not normally aware. In this stage primary modes of thought predominate and there is the emergence of visual imagery, symbolism, a kind of timelessness, and the absence of the usual logic. In a sense the patient knows a great deal about his problem, but he prefers to phrase it for himself and in therapy to communicate it at a symbolic level. The hypnotic relationship becomes a relatively safe place to experience the anxiety surrounding his neurotic conflicts symbolically and to work through the implications of these symbols in real life.

Most of these highly connotative symbols deal directly with either interpersonal relationships (including the relation with the therapist), or with aspects of one's self. Time and again the patient is placed in situations where he has a choice of whether or not to confront his problem at a symbolic level. Usually he expresses a willingness to do so because, for the first time, he is in company with someone he trusts and in whom he has confidence. Hypnosis automatically increases the status and prestige of the hypnotist, as witnessed objectively in the use of hypnosis to alter certain social stereotypes (see Chapter Five). In a very real sense, the patient engages in an elaborate role-playing or psychodrama in his dreams (or hypnoprojective fantasies), but the difference is that at the moment his dreams are completely real to him. In this manner, the therapist attempts to re-educate the patient in relation to his own personal, affect-laden images. To put it another way, dreams really are "the royal road to the unconscious," since symbols, as was stated earlier, contain a great deal of emotional imagery — there is no such thing as a neutral symbol. When you deal with a patient's symbols you deal with highly charged affective meaning.

What has been said is not intended in any way to derogate the clinical sagacity of the therapist. Obviously anyone can learn to hypnotize with very little practice and the success of hypnosymbolic treatment depends very much on the skilled therapeutic techniques of the clinician. The point is that while the therapist is *directive* in structuring the situation in which symbols can be produced, he becomes *nondirective* in attempting either to produce the specific symbols or to interpret them. He then becomes *relatively directive* again in attempting to relate the interpreted symbols to present problems and eventually to resolve some major portion of the client's conflict in a relatively short period of time. The therapist throughout stresses a warm, permissive, nonevaluative atmosphere which encourages free expression from the patient.

As was stated in "Brief Crisis-Oriented Hypnotherapy" (Moss, 1967a):

Only the predisposition to view hypnosis in terms of the well-ingrained historical stereotype, including the widespread tendency to conceive of it as a physiologically determined state, prevents recognition that the hypnotic relationship is as malleable as any other therapeutic transaction. The nature of the relationship, including the specific hypnotic techniques used, will vary with the therapist's personality, training, and clinical competence, and most importantly, the special needs of the patient. The successful hypnotherapist knows that the hypnotized patient remains an individual with full rights and privileges whose wishes and needs must be constantly consulted and consistently respected. If the situation requires it, hypnotherapy can be a highly nondirective venture, at least in the sense that it is possible to provide patients with illuminating and convincing insight-producing experiences that largely obviate the need for direct interpretation.

. . . Specialized hypnotic techniques then provide the means whereby distorted perceptions and conceptions can be rapidly uncovered, ramifications traced, implications explored, and a re-evaluation effected in terms of present reality. Most authorities agree that to be effective, psychotherapy must be more than an intellectual exercise — it must be an "emotionally corrective experience." Brief hypnotherapy allows for a decisive, convincing confrontation with troublesome memories, attitudes, and feelings, and even one such experience can have a healthy catalytic effect on treatment, leading to an acceleration of the whole process (pp. 252–253).

Despite the emphasis on hypnotic techniques throughout this book, a great deal of time is actually spent in trying to merge the repressed content into the waking life of the patient. These experiences must be understood and their meaning adopted by the remainder of the personality. To put it another way, the person suffering from a behavior disorder displays an increased distance between the latent and manifest content and hypnosis partially reduces this distance, but the meaning of the symbolic expression must be integrated into the waking state. But at the same time, let us admit that a great deal of what goes on in hypnosymbolic treatment remains essentially unknown (or can only be guessed at) by the therapist. In the majority of instances, the therapist may be quite surprised by the meaning attributed to the symbols by the patient. Dreams in therapy are communications between the patient and his therapist, but more important, as Sacerdote emphasized in his book, *Induced Dreams* (1967), they are considered also to be a dialogue between the patient's conscious and unconscious thoughts of which the therapist may have, at times, only partial understanding. The best available evidence is needed to know how to proceed in the re-education of the patient; but in large measure, one also knows that a therapist is often only a humble participant-observer of what is going on in the patient.

THE RELATIONSHIP TO BEHAVIOR THERAPY

Visualization or the experiencing of images and metaphors in lieu of or in combination with verbal concepts exists in a great many different psychotherapies. It is certainly present in psychoanalysis, to say nothing of Jung's technique of "active imagination" (described by G. Adler, 1948). At earlier times it appeared in Happich's (1932) meditative psychotherapy or Desoille's *rêvé eveillé dirigé* (the guided waking daydream), or later in the initiated symbol projection method of Leuner (described by Swartley, 1965) or the better known meditative exercises of autogene training (Schultz, 1964). Still more recently it has appeared in various forms of so-called behavior therapy, such as the visualization aspect of desensitization (Wolpe, 1958), the technique of emotive imagery (Lazarus and Abramovitz, 1962), or the direct sensory experiences involved in implosive therapy (Stampfl and Levis, 1968).

The assumption in behavior therapy is that behavior can be altered by direct modification of specific responses. The behavior therapist specifies the defined behavior he wishes to modify and by studying the conditions which support it, he undertakes to alter the reinforcement that maintains the response and attempts to replace it by more acceptable behavior. The behavior therapist does not concern himself with postulated intermediating processes such as the "unconscious." The "unconscious" is a factor only to the extent that the person believes that potent forces outside of his awareness influence his behavior. The behavior therapist's assessment is clearly on the client's conscious report and he is against such things as projective devices which he considers to be superfluous. Be that as it may, it clearly seems to work with many children where the problem is clearly defined and where the environment is open to specific control, as well as with motivated adults who wish to alter specific symptoms. The danger of symptom substitution is apparently another tenet of psychoanalytic faith which is not borne out.

Behavior therapy has a relatively great acceptance of hypnosis, as long as one discards the theory that currently underlies hypnotherapy and hypnoanalysis (Ullmann and Krasner, 1969). Hypnosis is accepted as a special form of role-playing elicited by the demands emanating from the placebo of the therapist. In practice, hypnosis is simply another device for attention-focusing and is used in visualization and/or relaxation. There is not sufficient evidence from the behaviorist's point of view that hypnosis can be used to reliably uncover the etiological factors underlying a patient's behavior, and even if this were possible, "insight" would be unnecessary for the cure of the specific symptom.

The chapter on a phobic case ("Black Rover, Come Over!") was deliberately featured here because it fit a specific Pavlovian paradigm with a well worked out technique of treatment. Discussion of this case should help to distinguish between a hypnodynamic and behavioristic orientation. In a more complex case the differences would be much less apparent since a model for the more complicated case has not been established and the treatment would have been much less specific. Undoubtedly the behavior approach would have been to simply attempt to countercondition this person through systematic desensitization to her fear of dogs. Even if successful, this would have left untouched all of the distorted relationships starting with the patient's mother and concluding with the sensitive relation with her own young daughter.

It is true that a reconditioning procedure was worked out with the hallucinatory dog, but only as a *symbol* of the complex interpersonal relationships. Now, if one accepts that in this case the dog really represented what the patient said it did, is the social learning theory of phobic behavior still correct in assuming that phobias are only conditioned fears? What would one say about the "little white dog" which plagued Alice's nightmares? The point is that the typical behaviorist often is not concerned about going into the patient's problems deeply enough to pinpoint the choice of the symptom or what really supports it. In this regard, it appears to be unnecessary in hypnotherapy to construct an elaborate anxiety hierarchy and to laboriously go over parallel experiences in successive approximations of the original trauma to desensitize the patient. In a very real sense, the patient sets his own stages in an informal hierarchy. (From the viewpoint of the therapist, one could also say that the treatment is much more interesting or much less boring than the behaviorist's methods.)

In such a patient his dreams, fantasies, and other projective productions constitute an internal representation of his conflict. The fact that he still produces such symbols attests to their current importance to him — they still describe a problem. Sometimes it is necessary to go back to the original choice of symbols, but in every instance the therapist rather quickly returns to the consequences of these symbols for the patient's present adjustment. In brief psychotherapy it is always necessary to be more concerned with the precipitating (recent) events than the predisposing ones (historical and childhood antecedents). The question is, what are the motivating factors that still sustain the neurotic symptoms? It must be acknowledged that hypnosymbolic therapy in this respect bears some resemblance to behavior therapy. Whereas the behavior therapist attempts to desensitize the patient's symptoms by structuring a reconditioning procedure which protects the patient as far as possible from the experience of any anxiety (Paul, 1968a, 1968b), the hypnotherapist first engages in a diagnostic procedure to attempt to determine the original situation that gave rise to the symptom; this situation is, of course, often fraught with anxiety. But once the hypnotherapist has a reasonably good idea of how the symptom was chosen, what it represents, and how it is sustained, then he attempts to structure a therapeutic situation that will also desensitize the patient to the full range of what the symptom represents at both conscious and unconscious levels.

At the same time, the dynamic and behavior practices are quite complementary: the virtue of providing "insight" into how a maladjusted behavior was learned is that it provides the client with added motivation to change, reduces resistances, and also provides precise information on the value of a planned behavior schedule in training *how* to change in a desired direction. It is not really a question of whether attitude changes cause a change in behavior or whether an alteration in perception precedes a change in behavior — both things should go on simultaneously. During the past few years the benefit of initiating desired behavior and having it followed by positive consequences so that the behavior will be maintained has been emphasized; in turn, the behavior therapists should also become aware of the necessity of looking at the human individual as a whole (past and present), of the importance of the meaning of events not overtly related to the problem behavior, and of the complexity of human behavior.

ARE THE SYMBOLS OBJECTIVELY VALID?

The dreams related in this casebook are almost always spontaneous nocturnal products or fantasies produced in the hypnotic situation itself, but in either case it is preferred to characterize them in the last analysis as projective content. The dreamer is always aware that his dreams and fantasies will be used in treatment. One cannot pretend that even night dreams (not a product of posthypnotic suggestion) are *pure* dreams uncontaminated by psychotherapy. Most dreams collected through electrophysiological (REM) laboratory studies are generally clear, coherent, believable occurrences of realistic situations in which the dreamer is involved in quite mundane and pedestrian pursuits (Snyder, 1967). In contrast, dreams presented to the therapist are rich, vivid, and complex — they provide the patient with an auxiliary form of communication with the therapist, allowing him to speak of things that he is not yet ready to commit to conventional language even to himself. The patient's dreams, tailored to the specific subject, reveal a great deal about the personality to the clinician, but at this juncture one must still say that he is dealing with projective fantasy produced either in the waking or sleeping state rather than saying that he is dealing with dreaming per se. This is a very thin line, but it comes from recognizing that the dreams presented to the clinician differ dramatically from the typical Stage 1–REM product. Even if the dreamer were outfitted with the usual electronic gadgetry and the dreams were collected throughout the night, one still could not be certain that he wasn't responding in terms of his expectations or the indirect suggestions that he received during the therapy hour. In this sense, training as a researcher perhaps gets in the way of functioning as an efficient clinician.

In the cases presented here, is the interpretative content elicited under hypnosis as to the meaning of the symbols actually valid in any objective sense? Were the subjects simply playing a role? Did the implicit social demands from the therapist force them to fabricate the clinical material that came forth? It is difficult to conceive that they made it all up, that it was an exercise of their creative imaginations which came about because they were "hypersuggestible." Through the employment of hypnosis the patients were able to present convincing causal connections between their various symptoms and earlier, traumatic experiences, often taken from early childhood. The connections revealed a precise, detailed, and convincing set of circumstances, and the symptoms have specific meaning which becomes transparently clear when the etiology is known. If one is familiar with the literature, then he will immediately know that this is a paraphrase of some of Joseph Breuer's comments he made over 75 years ago in the celebrated "Case of Anna." The reports of these patients are as convincing as Breuer and Freud (1950) found in their early studies. This author is an eclectic, not a psychoanalyst; he picks and chooses from all orientations and is a pragmatist, being guided by the results. He is also a reasonably objective observer, a researcher who tends to be skeptical about most everything (including hypnotism). Consider the dreams and fantasies given by José and Alice. Even today the therapist is somewhat shocked and put a bit off balance when an occasional patient's content appears to confirm Freudian theory, because it is unexpected and nothing is consciously done to demand it.

Most of these cases, of course, did not reveal predominantly sexual symbols and the data clearly imply that anything like universal symbolism remains unsubstantiated. The process of symbolism confronts the clinician with a complex and uncertain subject matter, and undoubtedly there is appeal in the closure provided by the comprehensive scope of orthodox psychoanalytic theory. However, this tendency toward clever, dogmatic speculations, far removed from objective, behavioral observations, is obviously not subscribed to here. The most that can be claimed is a universality of the evaluation-potency-activity affective meaning basis.

It is also anticipated that many psychotherapists who are devotees of extended treatment designed to effect basic alterations of character might argue that the interpretations or projections assigned by the patient are relatively superficial. Admittedly, the focus of treatment is ahistorical, on the here-and-now of current reality problems. This therapist has no doubt that if he had imposed a demand for another type of content, the patients probably would have acquiesced in their dreams and/or interpretations. Obviously, dreams are susceptible to different levels of interpretation; however, in the final analysis an interpretation is legitimate in the therapy situation only when it "means" something and is useful to the patient. An interpretation may be theoretically correct but psychologically wrong in its timing. It is felt that the criterion of meaningfulness was met with these patients when, through the use of hypnosis, they were able to render interpretations of their own dream productions which were then transformed into effective action in immediate problem situations.

There can never be an absolute, completely objective validation of what any dream actually means, but even if the patient's interpretations of his dreams are accepted only as extremely rich projective material, they prove of great value in the conduct of psychotherapy.

Success or failure of these techniques will partly be determined by the particular proficiency of a therapist in dealing with specific disorders; when used in the manner described, the hypnosymbolic method has many applications, including the provocation of rather spectacular graphic portrayals of defensive maneuvering. The author was once assigned a Negro patient hospitalized for 14 years as "criminally insane" because of the murder of his girlfriend with an ice pick. He had persistently claimed amnesia for the three-day period surrounding the event. He had made a model hospital adjustment and the chief psychiatrist was willing to consider his discharge, but he first requested that hypnosis be used in an effort to recapture the original event. The patient appeared to be a cooperative hypnotic subject and two sessions of conversation narrowed the period of amnesia to within 15 minutes of the assault; however, he stubbornly maintained that he had no memory for the actual attack. The patient under hypnosis was requested to visualize a book said to contain the long-avoided "insight." He was told that a breeze would riffle the pages and when it stopped, the book would remain open at a page containing a paragraph describing the disavowed incident. The patient dutifully reported seeing the book and the fluttering pages, but when instructed to read the paragraph, he insisted that a sheet of onionskin obliterated the words. When this obstacle was suggested away, he reported that the print was too fine to read, and when it was "magnified," the significant passage was found to be written in "mysterious hieroglyphics." A few such episodes drive home the point that resistances may be reduced in the hypnotic relationship, but they are not removed, and the ingenuity of the diagnostician using hypnosis in counteracting such defensive tactics is often sorely taxed.

BACK TO COMMUNITY MENTAL HEALTH

In this day of rapidly developing community mental health programs, with the realistic expectation that within a decade or two several thousand comprehensive mental health centers will be built, it is hoped that the change in location of mental health services will also be accompanied by very definite alterations in practice. The principal assumption underlying the whole proposed national mental health program is that the majority of mentally ill persons can be successfully treated in their own communities and quickly returned to useful roles in society, without prolonged treatment in the traditional custodial public hospital. The key concept in this program is *continuity of care* in the patient's home community. It is clearly intended that the program of services be available to *all* persons without respect to race, color, creed, or the ability to pay, nor shall persons be excluded from treatment on the basis that they do not meet a requirement of residence in such an area; these services will be provided to patients of all ages, both sexes, and without regard to diagnostic classification, including chronicity. In other words, ideally this program is intended to provide high-quality mental health care for everyone.

In the past, most community agencies and clinics carefully selected their patients on the basis of aptitude for certain specialized forms of treatment. Large numbers of patients were excluded on grounds of the kind of illness, limited education or verbal facility, level of income, and so forth. In contrast, the comprehensive community mental health center must be prepared to treat patients without regard to the nature or degree of dysfunctioning. Ideally, patients will no longer be fitted into a treatment pigeonhole; instead, treatment will be tailored to meet the particular patient's needs. As the program expands to meet the health needs of everyone, the professional manpower shortage will become increasingly acute.

It appears that extensive individual psychotherapy, with its preoccupation with intrapsychic dynamics, will become largely passé. "Talking therapies" will be largely restricted to brief, crisis-oriented sessions focused on the resolution of immediate reality-oriented problems, not unlike the suicide prevention programs developing throughout the country. Mental health professionals will increasingly have the prerogative of direct intervention in a patient's life and they will engage in environmental manipulations in a manner conducive to his mental health. The patient will be treated in the context of his family and his neighborhood. Social treatment, of course, will be combined with increasingly sophisticated applications of chemotherapy.

This particular form of hypnosymbolic treatment is prompt, focused, and reality-oriented. It acts to free the fantasy and imagination, allowing access to preconscious and unconscious content; it encourages memorial reversion, so that patients can move flexibly along the time continuum, living and re-experiencing the past and comparing and contrasting the past with present perceptions. The intensity of mental imagery solicited through hypnosis encourages a direct reconditioning process. These experiences are both revelationary and convincing. It need not be limited to persons who are temperamentally introspective, verbally fluent, and who can think conceptually. Research remains to establish how far it can be effectively used with persons of limited intelligence and schooling, that is, persons who are culturally, socially, or even innately deprived.

REFERENCES

Adler, G. 1948. *Studies in analytical psychology*. London: Routledge and Kegan Paul.

Alexander, F. 1929. *The psychoanalysis of the total personality*. Monograph No. 52. New York: Nervous and Mental Disease Publ. Co.

Alexander, F., and French, T. M. 1946. *Psychoanalytic therapy*. New York: Ronald Press.

Allport, G. W. 1954. *The nature of prejudice*. Cambridge, Mass.: Addison-Wesley.

Aumack, L. 1957. The Szondi: internal or external validation? *Perceptual and Motor Skills*, 7:7–15.

Bellak, L., and Small, L. 1965. *Emergency psychotherapy and brief psychotherapy*. New York: Grune and Stratton.

Borstelmann, L. J., and Klopfer, W. G. 1953. The Szondi Test: a review and critical evaluation. *Psychological Bulletin*, 50:112–132.

Brenman, M. 1949. Dreams and hypnosis. *Psychoanalytic Quarterly*, 18:455–465.

Breuer, J., and Freud, S. 1950. *Studies in hysteria*. A. A. Brill, trans. Boston: Beacon Press.

Buros, O. (Ed.) 1953. *The fourth mental measurements yearbook*. Highland Park, N.J.: Gryphon Press.

―――. 1959. *The fifth mental measurements yearbook*. Highland Park, N.J.: Gryphon Press.

―――. 1965. *The sixth mental measurements yearbook*. Highland Park, N.J.: Gryphon Press.

Caplan, G. 1964. *Principles of preventive psychiatry*. New York: Basic Books.

Cheek, D. B. 1959. Perception of meaningful sounds during surgical anesthesia as revealed under hypnosis. *American Journal of Clinical Hypnosis*, 1:101–113.

————. 1964. Surgical memory and reaction to careless conversation. *American Journal of Clinical Hypnosis*, 3:237–239.

Deri, S. 1949. *Introduction to the Szondi Test, theory and practice.* New York: Grune and Stratton.

————. 1952. In D. Brower and L. Abt (Eds.), *Progress in clinical psychology.* New York: Grune and Stratton.

Desoille, R. 1945. *Le rêvé eveillé en psychotherapie.* Paris: Presses Universitaires de France.

Erickson, M. H. 1935. A study of an experimental neurosis hypnotically induced in a case of ejaculatio praecox. *British Journal of Medical Psychology*, 15:34–50.

————. 1944. The method employed to formulate a complex story for the induction of an experimental neurosis in a hypnotic subject. *Journal of General Psychology*, 31:67–84.

Erickson, M. H., and Kubie, L. 1938. The use of automatic drawing in the interpretation and relief of a state of acute obsessional depression. *Psychoanalytic Quarterly*, 7:95–133.

————. 1940. The translation of cryptic automatic writing of one hypnotic subject by another in a trance-like dissociated state. *Psychoanalytic Quarterly*, 9:51–63.

Farber, L., and Fisher, C. 1943. An experimental approach to dream psychology through the use of hypnosis. *Psychoanalytic Quarterly*, 12:202–216.

Forer, B. R., et al. 1961. Custom-built projective methods: a symposium. *Journal of Projective Techniques*, 25:3–31.

Frank, J. D. 1961. *Persuasion and healing: a comparative study of psychotherapy.* Baltimore: Johns Hopkins University Press.

Freud, S. 1952. *On dreams.* James Strachey, trans. New York: W. W. Norton.

————. 1953. *A general introduction to psychoanalysis.* Joan Riviere, trans. New York: Permabooks, Doubleday.

————. 1960. *The interpretation of dreams.* James Strachey, trans. New York: Basic Books.

————. 1963. *An autobiographical study.* James Strachey, trans. New York: W. W. Norton.

Friedlander, J. W., and Sarbin, T. 1938. The depth of hypnosis. *Journal of Abnormal and Social Psychology*, 33:281–294.

Fromm, E. 1951. *The forgotten language.* New York: Rineland.

Gill, M. M., and Brenman, M. 1959. *Hypnosis and related states: psychoanalytic studies in regression.* New York: International University Press.

Guertin, W. H., and McMahan, H. G. 1951. A survey of Szondi research. *American Journal of Psychiatry,* 108:180–184.

Guido, J. A., and Jones, J. 1960. "Placebo" (simulation) electroconvulsive therapy. *American Journal of Psychiatry,* 117:838–839.

Hall, C. S. 1948. Frequencies in certain categories of manifest content and their stability in a long dream series. *American Psychologist,* 3:274 (abstract).

———. 1966. A comparison of the dreams of four groups of hospitalized mental patients with each other and with a normal population. *Journal of Nervous and Mental Disease,* 143:135–139.

Hall, C. S., and Van de Castle, R. L. 1966. *The content analysis of dreams.* New York: Appleton-Century-Crofts.

Happich, C. 1932. Das Bildbewusstsein als ansatzstelle psychischer Behandlung. *Zentr. Psychotherapie,* vol. 5.

Harriman, P. L. 1943. New approach to multiple personalities. *American Journal of Orthopsychiatry,* 13:638–643.

Jones, E. 1950. *Papers on psychoanalysis.* 5th ed. London: Bailliere, Tindall and Cox.

Lazarus, A. A., and Abramovitz, A. 1962. The use of "emotive imagery" in the treatment of children's phobias. *Journal of Mental Science,* 108:191–195.

Luria, Z. 1959. A semantic analysis of a normal and a neurotic therapy group. *Journal of Abnormal and Social Psychology,* 58:216–220.

McDowell, M. 1948. An abrupt cessation of major neurotic symptoms following an hypnotically induced artificial conflict. *Bulletin of Menninger Clinic,* 12 : 168–177.

Mazer, M. 1951. An experimental study of the hypnotic dream. *Psychiatry,* 14:265–277.

Miller, N. E. 1944. Experimental studies of conflict. In J. McV. Hunt (Ed.), *Personality and the behavior disorders.* New York: Ronald Press.

———. 1948. Theory and experiment relating psychoanalytic displacement to stimulus response generalization. *Journal of Abnormal and Social Psychology,* 43:155–178.

Moss, C. S. 1953. Quantitative semantic analysis of dreams in psychotherapy. Ph.D. thesis, University of Illinois.

————. 1957a. Dream symbols as disguises. *Etc.: Journal of General Semantics*, 14:267–273.

————. 1957b. A forced hypnoprojective fantasy used in the resolution of pseudoepileptic seizures. *Journal of Clinical and Experimental Hypnosis*, 5:59–66.

————. 1957c. Use of the schizophrenic in Rorschach content analysis. *Journal of Projective Techniques*, 21:384–390.

————. 1960a. Brief successful psychotherapy of a chronic phobic reaction. *Journal of Abnormal and Social Psychology*, 60:266–270.

————. 1960b. Current and projected status of semantic differential research. *Psychological Record*, 10:47–54.

————. 1960c. Dream symbols as disguises: a further investigation. *Etc.: Journal of General Semantics*, 18:217–226.

————. 1961. Experimental paradigms for the hypnotic investigation of dream symbolism. *International Journal of Clinical and Experimental Hypnosis*, 9:105–117.

————. 1965. *Hypnosis in perspective*. New York: Macmillan.

————. 1967a. Brief crisis-oriented hypnotherapy. In J. E. Gordon (Ed.), *Handbook of Clinical and experimental hypnosis*. New York: Macmillan, pp. 238–257.

————. 1967b. *The hypnotic investigation of dreams*. New York: John Wiley and Sons.

Moss, C. S., and Stachowiak, J. G. 1963. The ability of hypnotic subjects to interpret symbols. *Journal of Projective Techniques*, 27:92–97.

Mowrer, O. H. 1953. *Psychotherapy: theory and research*. New York: Ronald Press, pp. 532–535.

Orne, M. T. 1962a. Antisocial behavior and hypnosis. In G. H. Estabrooks (Ed.), *Hypnosis: current problems*. New York: Harper and Row, pp. 137–192.

————. 1962b. Hypnotically induced hallucinations. In J. D. West (Ed.), *Hallucinations*. New York: Grune and Stratton, pp. 211–219.

Osgood, C. E. 1953. *Method and theory in experimental psychology*. New York: Oxford University Press.

————. 1964. Semantic differential technique in the comparative study of cultures. *American Anthropology*, 66:171–199.

Osgood, C. E., and Luria, Z. 1954. A blind analysis of a case of multiple personality using the semantic differential. *Journal of Abnormal and Social Psychology*, 49:579–591.

Osgood, C. E., and Suci, G. J. 1952. A measure of relation determined by both mean difference and profile information. *Psychological Bulletin*, 49:251–262.

Osgood, C. E., Suci, G. J., and Tannenbaum, P. H. 1957. *The measurement of meaning*. Urbana: University of Illinois Press

Osgood, C. E., and Tannenbaum, P. H. 1955. The principle of congruity in the prediction of attitude change. *Psychological Review*, 62:42–55.

Packard, V. 1957. *The hidden persuaders*. New York: Cardinal.

Parad, H. J. (Ed.) 1965. *Crisis intervention: selected readings*. New York: Family Service Association of America.

Paul, G. L. 1968a. Outcome of systematic desensitization. I: Background, procedures and uncontrolled reports of individual treatment. In C. M. Franks (Ed.), *Assessment and status of the behavior therapies*. New York: McGraw-Hill.

———. 1968b. Outcome of systematic desensitization. II: Controlled investigations of individual treatment, technique variations, and current status. In C. M. Franks (Ed.), *Assessment and status of the behavior therapies*. New York: McGraw-Hill.

Phillips, E. L., and Wiener, D. N. 1966. *Short-term psychotherapy and structured behavior change*. New York: McGraw-Hill.

Rabin, A. I. 1950. Szondi's pictures: identification of diagnoses. *Journal of Abnormal and Social Psychology*, 45:392–395.

Rapaport, D. 1951. *Organization and pathology of thought* (Section III: Symbolism). New York: Columbia University Press.

Reeves, M. P. 1954. An application of the semantic differential to Thematic Apperception Test material. Ph.D. thesis, University of Illinois.

Regardie, F. I. 1950. Experimentally induced dreams of psychotherapeutic aids. *American Journal of Psychotherapy*, 4:643–650.

Sacerdote, P. 1967. *Induced dreams*. New York: Vantage Press.

Schafer, D. 1960. As-if electroshock therapy in hypnosis. *American Journal of Clinical Hypnosis*, 2:225–227.

Schultz, J. H. 1964. *Das autogene Training*. 11th German ed. Stuttgart: George Thieme Verlag.

Shaffe, H. 1953. A method for judging all contrasts in the analysis of variance. *Biometrika*, 40:87–104.

Snider, J. G., and Osgood, C. E. (Eds.) 1969. *Semantic differential technique: a source book*. Chicago: Aldine.

Snyder, F. 1967. The physiology of dreaming. In *Symposium on dream psychology and the new biology of dreaming*. University of Cincinnati.

Stachowiak, J. G., and Moss, C. S. 1965. Hypnotic alteration of social attitudes. *Journal of Personality and Social Psychology*, 2:77–83.

Stampfl, T. G., and Levis, D. J. 1968. Implosive therapy — a behavioral therapy? *Behavior Research and Therapy*, 6, no. 10: 31–36.

Swartley, W. 1965. Initiated symbol projection. In R. Assagioli (Ed.), *Psychosynthesis: a manual of principles and techniques*. New York: Hobbs, Dorman and Co., pp. 287–303.

Tostado, J. A. 1970. Ideational differences between suggestibles and nonsuggestibles as measured by the semantic differential. Master's thesis, University of Illinois.

Ullmann, L. P., and Krasner, L. 1969. *A psychological approach to abnormal behavior*. Englewood Cliffs, N.J.: Prentice-Hall.

Watkins, J. G. 1956. Projective hypnoanalysis. In L. M. LeCron (Ed.), *Experimental hypnosis*. New York: Macmillan, pp. 442–462.

Weitzenhoffer, A. M., and Hilgard, E. R. 1959. *Stanford Hypnotic Susceptibility Scale*. Palo Alto, Calif.: Consulting Psychologists Press.

Wolberg, L. E. (Ed.) 1965. *Short-term psychotherapy*. New York: Grune and Stratton.

Wolpe, J. 1958. *Psychotherapy by reciprocal inhibition*. Stanford, Calif.: Stanford University Press.

INDEX

A NOTE ON THE AUTHOR

C. Scott Moss is professor of psychology at the University of Illinois. He received his B.S. from the University of Wisconsin in 1948 and his Ph.D. from the University of Illinois in 1953. He subsequently filled a joint appointment as chief psychologist at State Hospital No. 1 in Fulton, Missouri, and associate professor of psychology at the University of Missouri. He also served as consultant to the Missouri state men's and women's prisons. In 1960 he was a visiting professor at the University of Kansas.

In 1961 he assumed the position of mental health consultant, National Institute of Mental Health (USPHS), Region IX, San Francisco, consulting on state and community mental health and related programs in the western United States (specializing in applied research and crime and delinquency). From 1965 to 1967 he was deputy to the associate regional health director for mental health services.

He has published numerous articles in his field. His two previously published books are *Hypnosis in Perspective* (1965), and *The Hypnotic Investigation of Dreams* (1967), which won the Society for Clinical and Experimental Hypnosis award for the best book of 1967 on hypnosis.

UNIVERSITY OF ILLINOIS PRESS